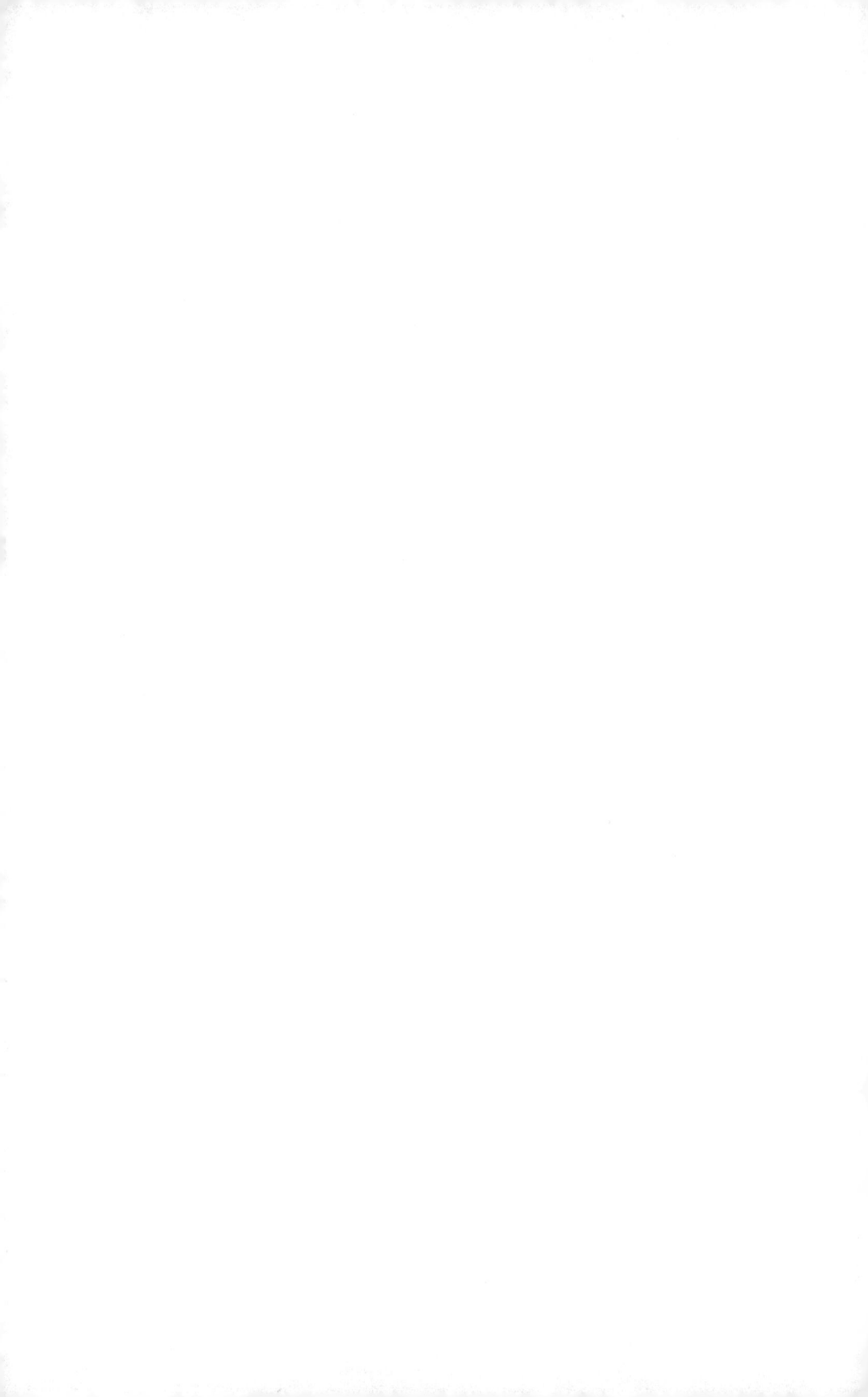

EXPERIENCE, STRENGTH, AND HOPE

MY RECOVERY FROM NICOTINE ADDICTION

1st Edition

GARY M.

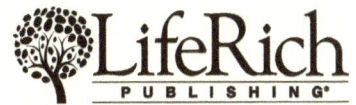

LifeRich Publishing is a registered trademark of The Reader's Digest Association, Inc.

LifeRich Publishing books may be ordered through booksellers or by contacting:

LifeRich Publishing
1663 Liberty Drive
Bloomington, IN 47403
www.liferichpublishing.com
844-686-9607

ISBN: 978-1-4897-3806-6 (sc)
ISBN: 978-1-4897-3805-9 (hc)
ISBN: 978-1-4897-3807-3 (e)

Library of Congress Control Number: 2021917698

Print information available on the last page.

LifeRich Publishing rev. date: 09/15/2021

CONTENTS

INTRODUCTION

Ol' PeaPickinWilly

Our Gary M. is a peach. He's got a great longtime quit going, he's silly and fun, and serious about working his program. And he models not taking ourselves too seriously—for us addicts who ride the drama rollercoaster. He is deeply involved in service work, both to Nicotine Anonymous World Service, and also in his home group, Voices of Nicotine Recovery. He keeps meetings lively and conversations about recovery stimulating. His stories ring true for many of us nicotine addicts, and his wisecrack jokes make recovery a whole lot more enjoyable.

These writings are a compilation of his shares on a Nicotine Anonymous (NicA) discussion forum and an email pen pal list. His insight from years of recovery has inspired many in their quest for reprieve from this insidious addiction.

This book is not about how to quit nicotine, rather it is one person's story about getting out of the prison of nicotine addiction, and his journey into a new life of enjoying freedom, feeling good, and being happy.

Aimee C.
cybrmavn
August 12, 2021

I am not writing about what you should do to quit your nicotine addiction but I am writing on how I did it. My quit date is Nov 21, 1998. It's about what I felt, what happened and where I am now. It was through this program of Nicotine Anonymous I was able to get some answers. I had finally after 49 years of smoking came to the conclusion I was completely powerless over this addiction and that I could not quit on my own. I smoked up to 4 packs a day and it almost took my life. I didn't quit a second too soon. What I have written in these various articles are my own opinions and how the steps worked in my life. Everything said here in written form are suggestions only. I cannot make you smoke, nor can I make you quit. That is your department. I hope and pray you get something out of what I wrote. All I can say is this all worked for me. There are other programs out there that have helped people quit but this is the only thing that worked for me.

A grateful addict

Gary M aka peapickinwilly
Aug 15th 2021

CHAPTER 1

EXPERIENCE

FEEL, DEAL AND HEAL

> Life in contented sobriety [smobriety] seems to be a matter
> of looking at the reality of myself in my attitudes, actions,
> and character rather than trying to run away from it.
>
> —AA Grapevine, September 2008

We had a topic in one of our online meetings which was "feel, deal, and heal." And this topic seems to fit that saying to a "T." I did not deal with feelings; I just pushed them deeper in my gut by smoking one more cigarette, one more pack, one more carton, week in and week out, month in and month out. It never ended. I was scared of my feelings and didn't know how to confront them. It was easier to numb them than deal with them. If I had to meet with someone over a touchy subject, I had to light up a cigarette, so I could stall before I said anything. When I got that feeling of being a victim, which was often, it felt good to smoke a cigarette to numb the feeling. I ran from my feelings, and I let the cigarette isolate me from them. And it was hell on wheels when I quit as all of a sudden these feelings jumped up at me by the zillions. Everyone around me got a piece of my action from my mouth. It worked overtime, and I stayed angry enough to feel justified in being angry. I mean like how dare they?

How I dealt with my feelings was an indication of what my attitude would be as I dealt with people, places, and things. My attitude was I felt I was basically a victim and I couldn't help myself. Everything that happened to me was the fault of others or circumstances. Yeah, there were some things I knew it was my doing, but my rationale on that was if they did what they did, I wouldn't have to do my bit. So, therefore, I shove the responsibility back to them. If I could ever get some decent breaks in life, I could be happy for a change. The only recourse I had in life was to smoke. I thought I was a happy camper as long as I had enough cigarettes on me at all times. All my actions, feelings, piss poor attitudes were all secondary as smoking was my primary objective. It was the only thing I could handle to adapt to life. And I thought it helped me. Little did I know what the truth was? I could not see living my life without a cigarette. Unconceivable! So I stayed on the angry side of life fighting the "good fight" ha!

As my character goes; it was full of defects, so consequently I really couldn't see anything good about myself. I really felt at times I was taking up space on this planet. Why am I here? Didn't have a clue but who cared as long as I had plenty of smokes. I could hide real easy under the umbrella of smoke and dream away in some stupid fantasy world that didn't exist.

I spent my life telling tall stories and embellishing the truth, stealing, was egotistical, was a thief, always behind in bill paying, justifying everything in sight. I was full of false pride and thought nothing of telling everyone how good I was and what I did and how I did it and brag and brag. I was selfish and lacked empathy for anyone. It was all about me.

So where did I go from here? I was sick and tired of smoking upwards to 4 packs a day and coughing my head off all the time. I was dizzy, hard to breathe and life was sucking me to death.

So we are at" feel, deal and heal." I had to know about my feelings before I could deal with them. The first thing I had to feel and deal with was quitting smoking. If I can't get to that point, then I will be stuck until I am willing to move forward through the steps and if I'm lucky, I won't die first. Nobody likes doing them. It becomes a matter of necessity to live that I did them, not because of what I am feeling physically or mentally or spiritually for that matter. It for me became an issue of living or dying. Two options only that I had to look at to decide what I wanted to do. I had to throw every excuse I had going for me out the window. Do I want to live or die! It's very elementary when you can get it to that point.

I'm powerless over nicotine, and now I move onto the fact that God can restore me to sanity. Now I ask myself, do I want to believe that God is and that He can restore me to sanity? The 2nd half of the First Step says that our lives had become unmanageable. Well, unmanageable equals insanity. They go hand in hand. I accept this step and now do I feel like I have been restored to sanity? No. It takes time. I have a ways to go yet. The Twelve Steps are like going to school for 12 years through High School. I am just at the 2nd grade level

But it's a start. Step Three "Made a decision to turn my life and will over to the care of God as I understand Him. Now, wait a minute you say, I have been doing pretty well by myself taking care of things. I don't need to trust something I cannot see and for what reason. I am doing okay. Oh Really!

Is that why I am always broke, in the hospital, sick as a dog, can't breathe, walking pneumonia, COPD, always angry, tired of people in my face all the time about my smoking. I am always looking for an answer besides quitting and spending over 15 years being a professional quitter. Give me a break. So what have I got to lose searching out this God? Is anybody going to see me get on my knees and pray? It gets back to the basics. Do I want to live or die? I smoke I- die, I quit-I live. Which is it? So I try to pray to this being which I call God and ask him simply just "help me." Pray for just today I do not smoke no matter what even if my ass falls off. At this point in my recovery I have become willing to surrender to God and whoever else I have to surrender to like a sponsor. Always keeping in mind do I want to live or do I want to die. I smoke one cigarette I am on my way to the gallows. There is no turning back.

I see my feelings pop up now left and right. I am angry, I am lonely, I am sad, I am scared, and these are feelings with having to learn to deal with them. The first thing is to try and find out why I am feeling these feelings. Don't run from the feeling, live and feel it. Look where it comes from. If I am fearful, then why? What am I scared of happening? Don't numb it, don't bury it, live with it and as you discover what causes it, then it will stop plaguing you. Fear is a basic emotion. If I hang on to that fear, then I get angry which is a defense mechanism for me. So it goes with being angry. Why am I angry? For all practical purposes, anger is based on fear of something. Deal with fear and the anger goes away.

What really helped me was to write a daily journal as to what I am feeling and why if I know, and why am I angry and what someone did to me. Or if I'm lonely, sad, makes no difference, just write it out and not worry about if you're right or wrong or worded just so—after all nobody is going to read it except you. I found this to be a huge benefit for me. It's a written history of my recovery. There have been times I felt I'm not getting anywhere. It's getting boring, or I'm wound up like a kite, and a cigarette seems so good. I read my journal, and after reading it, I see where my thinking is wrong. My brain anyhow has the amazing ability to forget what was bad but only remembers the "good" like how good a cigarette makes me relax. That's a joke! It forgets how my chest hurt from coughing waiting for one of my ribs to break or have a heart attack or laying on the floor and can't breathe. What all the steps do is help me feel and deal with myself, and in the process, the healing comes into play.

The Fourth Step Inventory was a major for me as I could see who I am not what I think I am or who I'm portraying to be for others to see. But the true me—the good, bad and ugly. Now that I can see it in written form I can learn to deal with it. I can see how I hurt people and what I need to do, I can begin to understand why I was always angry. Nothing pleased me. After I quit smoking, it didn't take long to be aware of how clean I smell. I used to be pure yellow in my fingers and stunk to high heaven. No wonder no one wanted to be around me. I can't stand to be around a smoker either. What goes around comes around. Doing my inventory, there were some good qualities about me, but at that stage of my life, I couldn't tell what was good or bad. That's one reason we take inventories, to clean house and get rid of the junk. So I put everything down on paper so I could look at the true person I was. It was hard to ascertain what was good or bad so I had to put everything on the shelf and let time take care of itself.

I wasn't all bad, but it was pretty bad. I learned that one good trait I had was commitment. If I said I was going to do something I would to my best and follow through. I tried not to cheat everyone and tried to be fair in my dealing with my customers etc.

Then there is the cop out step….ha-ha…Step Five—Admitted to God and another Human being the exact of nature of my wrongs. That's where you tell somebody about what you wrote about yourself. Now that person can be anybody. Your sponsor, a therapist, a minister, your spouse, a good friend, it doesn't matter who you read this stuff too, but the important thing is to do it and find somebody you can trust to keep their mouth quiet. This is in the spirit of anonymity. Now you can use one person or several, doesn't matter as long as you do it. Myself, I used my sponsor, my therapist, and my wife. Whatever works, works. Just don't leave anything out. If you do, you will pay for it down the road somewhere.

Now I was beginning to heal. I could see daylight much better at the end of the tunnel, and it was getting brighter. As I learn about myself and what I am, then I could ask God for help in restoring me to sanity.

I believe it says in our red book that sanity being restored begins at the 7th step and I believe this to be true. Before I could ask God for specifics in my recovery, I have to know what it is I am asking Him to help me. It stands to reason. How can I ask God or anybody for that matter for help if I do not know what help I need?

Now in the next two steps, I learn about my defects of character and shortcomings. This is interesting.

In the 5th step I am looking for the exact nature of my wrongs. In Step 6 was entirely ready for God to remove our defects of character, and in the 7th step asking him to remove our shortcomings.

Exact nature of my wrongs—was ready to remove our character defects—ask to remove our shortcomings. Is this the one and the same with a different name to it? I had heard that Bill W when he wrote up the 12 steps in AA that he didn't like to use the same word in each sentence. At first glance, I thought this sounds dumb, all three steps meaning the same thing. What's the point of doing that? One step should solve the problem. But Bill W was right. Here is the deal. Step Five we tell to another human being the exact nature of our wrongs, Step Six "Were entirely ready to have God remove all these defects of character" And in Step Seven "We humbly ask him to remove our shortcomings. So we have "exact nature of our wrongs, character defects, and last but least shortcoming. All are meaning the same thing but there is a different action to be taken in these three steps. Step five—we tell someone, Step Six—we become willing and Step Seven—we ask.

It's keeping it simple that counts. And once I started on my amends, it lifted many burdens from my shoulder not to mention resentments because for the most part in my "opinion" it was there doing that made me do what I did. And by making amends, I felt better as a person, and my attitude toward life changed. It healed a lot of issues with people I had hurt. My victim personality left me; I was more content as I had a purpose in life and what was that? Sharing my Experience, Strength, and Hope with everyone. That gave me a sense of well-being.

So feel, deal and heal is what we all are looking for or we wouldn't be here. I feel content with my life. I don't have everything I would like or the ability to go on vacations and things like that, but God gives me all my needs every day. And I am content with what I have, not what I don't have. Here is the one insane lie I believed all my life. Smoking was a good thing in my life. It made me feel good about myself, gave me courage, gave me substance in my life. Now that turned out to be a big fat lie…maybe at the beginning of my smoking career this might have been true but it turned on me very slowly over the years, so slow I couldn't see the elephant in the living room. And it almost took my life.

Now I have total freedom in not having to smoke and can do what I want with my life and not worry about smoking, just as long as I practice these principles in all my affairs. It was a long walk, but I am outta of that tunnel, and the sun shines. How about dem apples?

INTELLECT VS. EMOTIONS

> If intellect rules over emotion, the result is normality, but
> if emotions rule over intellect, the result is insanity.
>
> ~Unknown

It seemed when I was smoking I ran on emotions and every time I made a decision it came out wrong. Well, I won't say every time, but a major portion of my decision making abilities was fried with emotions. That set me up to run in an insane fashion. I would get discouraged and smoke over these lame decisions I made. There was no thought put behind them. Either it felt good, I was fearful, I was angry, I was depressed, and ad infinitum. And these emotions changed every few minutes. So how can I expect good results when my emotions were chaotic? So what did I do? Hell, I smoked myself into oblivion, that's what all good nicotine addicts do. Is that insane or what? Nothing rational, that's for sure. I gave it no thought especially if it "felt" like the right thing to do. Feelings change one minute to the next so you can see how your decisions are erratic as hell.

How about if your car is old but still running okay, has a few dents, needs some mechanical work and your low on money. When the emotions are running havoc on you, you think, shit we need a new car, it will be more pleasurable and won't be ashamed of having this old car while everyone else seems to have a nice car. So you talk yourself into buying a low price new car and wind up being talked up to a higher priced car, and the payments are higher than you want, and the car insurance goes up, so you kid yourself into signing the contract. After a down payment which you can't afford and maybe $350 a month payment for 36 months and you're only leasing it, and it will never be yours, but you can now travel in style. Believe me, the newness will wear off and the reality will hit you like a ton of bricks as to what you have done.

Now if the intellect rule over this decision, I would have weighed up the true costs, and what is the better way overall in the long run? I would have no car payments; my insurance would be lower. I know the condition of my car and see no heavy expenses. So it's beat up a bit, so what. I don't drive much anymore, and it's no big deal. Getting by on my low income and no car payment is a big deal. No one can repossess it as they tried once before as I got way behind in my payments. I have freedom from financial insecurity. I need more debt like a hole in the wall. This is insane thinking. The more times I work with my intellect rather than my emotion, I appreciate the freedom it gives me. Putting myself into a stressful condition by letting my emotions run helter- shelter puts me into danger of wanting a cigarette to escape the stress I put myself into harm's way. I look over my life, and I can see where most of the problems I am faced with are my own doing — usually caused by my emotions.

There are times I am tossed to and fro with a decision, and I don't know what to do. Usually, in these cases, I will wait until the time comes when I know that I know the answer is yes or the answer is no. Then and only then do I make a decision. Sometimes this is God's way of helping me make a good decision. It teaches me patience to wait on the Lord. There are times I flat out do not know what to do, so I pray and wait. "You don't need the ticket 'till the train gets here" I sometimes think God has a sense of humor and other times he wants me to wait, and I don't feel like waiting. It sure would help the stress level if I knew a few days in advance.... lol

Sometimes though, I get into the position a bad decision is better than no decision. If I make no decision, then I am paralyzed with fear and do nothing. So there are times, I have to do something even if it's wrong. If it's wrong, then I can make another decision until I get it right. It's like driving to a destination, and you're not sure which turn to make. So in those cases, make a left or right turn and see where it takes you. By process of elimination, you will get where you're going. However, the most logical decision is to pull over somewhere and ask where is such and such?

Then as it's been said' "He who hesitates is lost," which primarily means if you sit back and think about something too long, you will lose out. It's okay to give thought to something that could benefit you, like a business opportunity or a job that is offered to you, but can go by the wayside it you put it to sleep. Life is always full of decisions on a day to day basis. Bottom line is you don't have a clue what to do, then do something then let the chips fall where they fall. You can always pick up the chips and try again. Unfortunately, there is no perfect answer. It's a matter of praying, believing and then put something into play.

So what does this all have to do with smoking? A whole lot! It's our makeup that makes us smoke. Screw up and running in fear; I would smoke to burn the fear away. Of course, it didn't go away so I had to smoke another one and then another one and so on.

Years ago when I had my business, I was behind in my payroll taxes several thousand dollars. I was not good with finances. I always believed in getting what I want out of life if there was anything left I paid some of my bills. The IRS got shoved to the bottom of the heap. One day the IRS came into my shop as I was closing up and wanted to look at my customer's addresses and names and I let them for a few minutes. Fear got a hold of me, and I yanked everything out of the agent's hands and physically threw them out of my doors and locked it. They yelled at me that they would get me. I called a lawyer and made an appointment with him that night, and I went to the bank and drew all my money out so the IRS wouldn't get it and filed Chapter 13 bankruptcy that night. The IRS was informed that they couldn't touch me or my accounts. Well the IRS didn't let that faze them. I had lots of money on the books, and they went to the customers that they could get addresses and phone numbers and put a hold on them to paying me. That stopped me cold for about 30 days when they were told by the court to stop it. I smoked one cigarette after another through all of this insanity. Making all these decisions based on my emotions rather than my logical reason was insane.

Nothing changes if nothing changes. I had to change my whole way of doing things if I expected to have any semblance of sanity. I learned to have fear in God to restore me to sanity, and that took some time processing the steps to get there. I look back at my financial way of doing things, and I just shake my head. It was crazy, to say the least. I live on now about 20% of what I used to make, and I get by just great. I live day to day on a day to day basis, and it's great. All I had to change is everything…ha-ha-ha-ha. I can see what being a four pack a day smoker got me. Nada!

Life is good today after 22 and half years of being a non-smoker. Should have learned this a long time ago but its better late than never.

WHAT ARE THE REQUIREMENTS FOR JOINING NICOTINE ANONYMOUS?

> Tradition Three: The only requirement for Nicotine Anonymous membership is a desire to stop the use of nicotine.
>
> ~Nicotine Anonymous

In this tradition it doesn't say an honest desire, it says a desire. It can be a very weak desire, but if you have some desire to give up nicotine, this makes you a member. There are no dues to pay, No promises to be made, heck you can even still smoke. After all, you can smoke and have a desire to quit. If you're an addict, you can't quit, at least you think can't quit. As you get into the program, you will see you can quit. You can't smoke in meetings but you can go outside and have a smoke, and no one is going to say anything.

The first meeting I ever went to I was told I could smoke and still be able to go to a meeting, so I thought to myself, this is great. I went to the meeting, and I see no one smoking and no ashtrays, and that moment I felt I had been had. What a bummer. It didn't occur to me that smoking was not allowed in the meeting, but I could go outside and smoke. Ha-ha. No one will make you quit smoking. You could smoke for the rest of your life and still come to meetings. After all you still have the desire and that makes you a bona fide member.

We can lead you to the water, but you have to work to drink the water. And ways those are my thoughts on the subject.

LIVING LIFE ON LIFE'S TERMS

I went to an online NicA meeting this morning which was a good way to start my day off. It never fails to make me feel better. Waiting to get a call from my brother to say there is some work to be done. I never know from day to day when I will have something to do. I get my SS benefits tomorrow, and it's all spent as it is every month. Sure doesn't go far but rent gets paid and all that stuff. But God takes care of my needs and knowing that and having the faith He will provide takes a huge load off my shoulder. I think back to all the things I used to worry about, and 9 of 10 times it was all for naught. All it did was rob me of energy, my emotions went awry and spent a restless night in bed. So I have learned to not sweat the petty stuff, it's just not worth it.

Worry is a lack of faith that God of my understanding will not be there to take care of my needs. As I look back, He was always there. The money would come in strange ways, problems would be taken care of, and all I had to do was step out of the way and let it happen. Yes, I have to take a step in the action, praying for something and doing nothing about it, won't work. I believe in the adage "God helps those, who help themselves. I have to take the first step. I have to do what I can do to set things in motion and leave the results up to God. And the best part is I do not have to smoke to hide my fears. I can do life without smoking or even have thoughts of smoking

I took a day off writing this, and now the weather is getting hotter. In the next few days, it's going to reach the 90's and my A/C is not working and with me having COPD does make it uncomfortable. Supposedly the tech is supposed to be out any day; he is waiting on some parts that are ordered. Man, am I going to enjoy the cold again. Makes it hard to breathe normally but smoking won't make it better. This too shall pass. If I would smoke, it would never pass. Thank God I don't smoke today. I just take each day as it comes. What really feels exotic for me is that I never get a thought of smoking no matter what happens. The act of smoking just does not enter my mind anymore. That's the best gift I could have ever received. It's a miracle that I am still alive today 22 and half years later.

The first thing I had to learn was just not to smoke today no matter what even if my ass falls off. If it falls off then just have someone put it back on for you, pick yourself up and move on. If you have had a bad day but not smoke, then you really have had a good day. Some days are hard, but I have learned to make the best of it as I know that nothing stays the same. If my feelings get hurt and I feel sorry for myself and pick up a cigarette, I can guarantee you I will feel like death warmed over and have to start all over again. Feelings change from one moment to the next so to make a life threatening decision like picking up again is insane as hell. But for me to have to start over again is a no brainer. I do not have another quit in me, and I protect my quit with the same passion as trying to protect my right to smoke.

I wake up in the morning and just lay there and take in deep breathes of air, and that feels so good without coughing. Things I used to take for granted are a life gift being given back to me. I stay connected with NicA through meetings, service and sharing my ESH with anyone who needs it. It's like paying my life insurance premiums in advance. The 12 Steps of recovery are my life blood. I don't just talk about them; I do them. That's what makes the difference. Well, guess what just happened?

My A/C tech just called and said the parts came in and he will be right down. Praise the Lord! I am susceptible to heat when it starts to get into the 80's as it causes me breathing problems. Today I did use my oxygen bottle for a couple of hours, and that helped. Normally I just use it to sleep with and that in itself is a blessing as I wake up with more energy and sleep well and fall asleep faster.

I don't look at myself as a victim because I have COPD caused you to know why? I got it by smoking, but I have learned to live with it. Having COPD is a fact and cannot be changed so why not just see what I can with my health to make it better. As long as it's cool and the humidity is low, I do quite well. I can't really exert myself, or I will be gasping for breath, and It doesn't bother me to let my brother, for example, change my welding bottles at work as there too heavy for me to handle nor do I try to be superman and lift things while knowing what the outcome will be by doing so. The hell with my pride, I can ask for help when needed. I have learned to slow down when working and amazing as it seems I still get my work done in a reasonable amount of time. My brother has A/C at work, and I have all the luxuries there I need. I have a refrigerator, microwave, a bed to sleep on if I want to stay overnight. And I can name my own hours. I can come and go as I please.

I guess what I am trying to say is one has to learn to live life on life's terms. And I'm constantly learning to do that. I do moan and groan at times, but it doesn't do me any good unless I put action behind it. Meaning if there is something I can do to alleviate the problem then I will and then accept the outcome.

If I can't do anything else to fix the problem, then I have to recognize it as the problem that became a fact — so knowing that I move on to the next problem. There is always a problem in the works just waiting for you. I have to learn to flow with things as they happen. I may not like it changing in mid-stream, but there are times I just have to do it—so I set my mind frame just to do what I have to do rather than fight it. It's so much easier to accept things in life than fight it. It gets my nerves jangled up, and I'm getting too old to set the world on fire anymore, not that I ever solved anything that way or not but it always had my adrenaline going, and I smoked one cigarette after another and that made matters worse as it got my adrenaline moving that much faster. So it really didn't calm me down. About all it did was to satisfy a craving.

I wake up in the morning praying to God for my smobriety and sobriety and help me through the day. And I talk to God throughout the day a word here and a word there, and it makes all the difference in the world. I just did some deep breathing, and that felt good. It sure takes the tenseness out of your body. And I didn't hear any wheezing or gurgling or a need to cough or anything like that. It feels so good not to smoke anymore. Or to put it more correctly, just not for today. I enjoy my life and enjoy living. I don't like a lot of things in life but who says you have to. I would be abnormal as hell if I liked everything. The things I don't like I have just had to leave it be and accept it as it is. I learn to keep my side of the street clean and learn to be grateful.

Some of you who are still struggling to get a stable quit, I can say it will change if you keep this to one day at a time, pray, go to meetings, stay in contact with other addicts, and this keeps your mind focused on your recovery. It will get better as long as you do the things necessary to protect your quit. This is not a program of thou shall not's, rather a program of what I need to do. For me, that is working the steps. And you don't do this one time; it is a life time process of doing and redoing. What NicA promises is good health and ways to stay quit contentedly. It does not necessarily mean your finances will improve; your marriage will get better, get better jobs or anything else. It just promises you a way out of this addiction. Yes in all likelihood other things in life will get better, but you may need to seek outside help to acquire what you need. And there is nothing wrong with that. As the old saying goes, "You don't go to a dentist to get legal advice" So you don't go to this program to get legal advice. You go to an attorney for that. You go to NicA to learn how to quit smoking. That is a big chore in itself.

That first year of quitting was really hard for me, and that is a very normal thing. I'm glad I went through what I did as it stays with me and it's as fresh as a new borne babe. I never want to forget where I came from.

I was "born" on Nov 21, 1998, and anything else before that was a prelude as for how smoking can kill me. And it almost did. I would have been dead in a couple of weeks to a month if I didn't quit when I did. I can picture myself so clearly in my final days of smoking and even then going to NicA I was a fighter, not willing to give up ideas of quitting which never worked but I had to hang onto my "pride" as it was all I had and that is not saying much at all. Surrender to me was a sign of weakness. But the paradox is if I gave into the concepts I was being taught, I would learn more and have a better life being nicotine free. But I couldn't envision a life without smoking. At the time it was non-negotiable. I wanted to quit but on my terms and I was looking for a way of quitting without quitting smoking. That statement in itself qualifies me for Step Two... lol

That was then, and this is now. I have been clean of nicotine for 22 years, seven months and six days. This was done one day a time. I deleted the word forever out of my mouth as forever never worked. I put my faith into God, worked the steps, got into service and made myself available when I can. I love this way of life, and it can be yours too....so go for it!

Gary M.

THE PRICELESS SECRET OF DAILY LIVING

> If you can take your troubles as they come, if you can maintain your calm and composure amid pressing duties and unending engagements, if you can rise above the distressing and disturbing circumstances in which you are set down, you have discovered a priceless secret of daily living. Even if you are forced to go through life weighed down by some inescapable misfortune or handicap and yet live each day as it comes with poise and peace of mind, you have succeeded where most people have failed. You have wrought a greater achievement than a person who rules a nation. Have I achieved poise and peace of mind?
>
> ~AA 24 Hour Thought for today

These are lofty goals to work toward achieving. Are they impossible? I don't think so. It is if you want perfection, but anything between a chaotic life style and a serene lifestyle is a good thing. I myself like to think I have reached near this life style. For the most part, I don't let things bother me to the point I am ready to kill or set the world of fire.

Before I ever worked the steps of this program, I was a very angry person and felt life was doing me a bad turn. Smoking was one way of dealing with life. I could bury the thoughts by smoking — one cigarette after another. I lived under the illusion; as long as I could smoke I could handle life. You talk about denial. Ha! I thought I could handle things even though I was angry all the time. I thought I had a right to be angry as life kept picking at me like I was the victim. Smoking gave me time to sit and meditate while swirling all the smoke in the air and I would come up with all kinds of lofty plans to solve my problems. And none of them worked. My solutions were built on deception so it was a given I would fail.

A lot of times I woke up with these ideas and didn't follow through with them as they appeared to me as being dumb at that point.

Through the process of putting these steps in my life, I have found for me I could deal with problems much better than I ever had before. The Steps taught me about myself as well as learning how to live a day at a time. That was a new way to live. If I was going to learn how to live a day at a time, then I had to be ready for some changes. All I had to do is change everything about myself. Which I might add was no easy chore but a very rewarding experience.

Just not smoking was a huge change, and I knew deep down just not smoking wasn't going to get it. I couldn't deal with life, and I couldn't deal with smoking any more. So the day came when I quit and had made up my mind "enough is enough" If I smoke one more cigarette it's going to kill me. At this point, I was desperate to try anything not to smoke. Ergo, the Steps. I was able to accept Step One and Step Two and Three weren't bad as I already understood who God was in my life, I just was pissed at Him as He couldn't get me to quit smoking. I didn't really have a problem with Step Four except it was too much work, so I didn't want to do it. Besides Step Five was the stopping point. I am not going to tell some other clown the "exact nature of my wrongs." I will be damned if I will do that. Lol. So, as long as I didn't do step 4, then I didn't have to worry about Step 5, and I stayed smober on the first three steps for the first year.

At the beginning, in my 2nd year I was a little unsettled as things were starting to return to where they were when I first quit smoking. I needed to move forward and these steps as they were suggested to me. And away I went, and it was really good for me to do that. I found out so many things about myself, and why I did them, it was truly amazing. God started to restore me to sanity, and this couldn't happen until I understood what my insanity issues were. Ergo, the steps. It's like taking your car to a mechanic to fix your car, and he asks what's wrong with it? I don't know just fix it. Right! The same thing goes with my internal thinking and emotional problems. I have to know what they are and what I need fixing before I can ask God to fix me.

After I began to get some clarity back into my life, I realized I was living life without really thinking about smoking. A few months after my first year being smober, the obsession to smoke finally for the most part disappeared. What a good feeling that turned out to be. Through the process of applying the steps in my life, I have become a different person or should I say the same person but a different attitude and a new take on life as well as really liking myself. What used to throw me for a loop I take in stride these days.

I have learned to be responsible for my own actions, which means if I am wrong, own up to it and if need be, correct it. I don't have to be right all the time, in fact, many times I have learned my thinking was wrong just by listening to other comments and keeping my mouth shut. "Be quick to listen, slow to speak" a verse in the Bible that fits quite well in my recovery. Engage your brain before you speak. I can't tell you how many times I opened up my mouth to put my two cents and had no idea what I was talking about and wound up looking like a fool. Say there is a serious discussion somewhere, I try to keep my thoughts to myself until all is said, and I can piece together my thoughts in a collective manner. If someone sends me an email or I am upset over what someone said I would get that email out faster than a bullet in retaliation. Lol. I sure got tired of eating crow. Now before I speak back in times like those intense moments, I wait a good 24 hours for me to cool off. I can put my email in a draft, and when I read it the next day, most of the time I said OMG, I'm glad I didn't send this.

When I have a problem to deal with, I try to find a solution for it and go for it. To do nothing and bitch about it gets me nowhere. If I can't come up with a concrete idea, then I turn it over to God for help. Then I forget about it and move on to another thing I need to do. By turning over to God, it really frees me up to do things I can do. In times of old,

I would be trying to fix everything and be overwhelmed with it all and would escape into a cigarette. That was my escape hatch. And smoking didn't fix anything either.

By asking God's help with my problems and having the faith God will answer, I can go on with the rest of my life and not worry about things where I have asked God's help. Worry ceases to really be a problem for me anymore. I have found over time worry is useless as I have no control over what happens. What I worry about is essentially lack of faith and most things I worry about don't come to pass. Now there is nothing wrong with worry. Let's say I'm worried about someone in the family who has a major health issue. Of course, I am worried about the outcome, but it really shows concern. If I didn't worry about those things, it doesn't say much about me. True I still give my concerns to God as there is nothing I can do. And that is what I should do.

So all this comes down to living one day at a time. It's a daily habit these days and staying in the day makes life so much simpler. As a way of life, I find I don't regret the past nor am I too concerned about the future. Yes, I make plans for the future, like doctor's appointments, when I have to work, when a bill is due when I am going somewhere and that's the way it should be. If I didn't make plans, I would be like a blind man walking not knowing where he is going. Now how those things work out is God's worry not mine. If it doesn't come to pass, well I will redo it and go on from there. I have pretty much concluded, nothing is really set in stone. For the most part there is nothing set as a deadline. There is always for the most part room for negotiating. Deadlines, for the most part, are put into place for scare tactics. But then again there are tickets, fines, court dates, etc. This shows there are exceptions to every rule.

I learn to accept things as they happen to the best of my ability. One reason I make it a goal of getting a good night's sleep. I can pretty much deal with what is thrown at me if I am feeling rested. Heaven forbid if I am tired....Shame on you! Ha-ha. I am like Dr. Jekyll and Mr. Hyde –like night and day. Kidding aside even when I am tired I do try and accept things as they are. Though I am apt to fail off and on, but that's being human. I live by the serenity prayer and focus it into my life.

Step Ten: "Continue to take a daily inventory and when we are wrong promptly admit it." As the day progresses, I have to be on the alert when I might say or do something that is wrong or perceived as wrong by others and try make an amend promptly. At the beginning that meant to me, when I get around to it, maybe next week or so, or when I am led to do so. Promptly means like before the day ends. "Don't let the sun go down over your anger" By me going to bed being angry or not taking care of something I will have disrupted my sleeping and also will bring about how I start the next day off. It becomes a way of life that for the most part a sense of well-being. There have been many instances I literally refuse to be angry over something. It's just not worth the frustration and anxiety it brings upon me.

So yes I can live in a peaceful mode for the most part and let things happen as they happen to realize I can't change circumstances. They are what they are. I put my trust into God as I understand Him and that is a miracle to me. I used to fantasize how nice it would be to live somewhere else where the grass is greener. The trouble is I have to bring myself to that greener paradise, and when I get there, I find the grass has lots of brown spots in it. So I have to change, so I can accept myself for who I am and be content with what I have and, not what I don't have. That is mandatory for me. And that is the name of that tune.

GRATITUDE AND THE MIRACLES OF RECOVERY

I'd like to talk about the things I am grateful for since I quit smoking. First of all, I am grateful that I have gained 22 years of my life by not smoking. I would have truly been dead within about two weeks if I didn't quit when I did.

My lungs were so black that the doctors couldn't tell what I had in them. The lights went out in my lungs. After a year light snuck in and then the doctor saw something he didn't like and I had to get a lung biopsy. Praise God; it turned out to be just scar tissue. It's amazing with all the smoking I did for 49 years. I was smoking four packs a day in my latter years of having "fun" and enjoying smoking. Ha!

In the last 22 years, I have been going through health problems. I've gone through bouts of kidney stones, kidney infections, living in a nursing home for a month, TIA stroke, arthritis, difficulties breathing and all the usual stuff that happens as we age. I am now on oxygen and have been for a year or so, and it's a blessing. I can breathe again and do things I wasn't able to. I can still work though it's tough at times, but I like staying active. I have emphysema which is incurable, and I accept that and probably will die from some form of lung problems.

The benefits I gained from smoking…lol, but the fact remains I am still alive and able to enjoy living one day at a time. Like I said if I didn't quit when I did I wouldn't be here writing to you all.

I never saved any money for retirement as I always believed in easy come, easy goes and I can do this forever… what a fool. Now I am paying for it. Now I am living on the other side of the financial spectrum. Somewhat poverty—low income, need to work to supplement my fixed income. Over the years I have adjusted to the fact I have to live within my means, and now it's fun. I can be happy and content and not have a dollar in my pocket. God does provide on a daily basis. I get food stamps, lower utility bills, a new refrigerator from my electrical company to save on energy. We are living in a cottage with 6 other neighbors with a cottage, and it's small with a garage. And because of a lawsuit waged against the LA airport for noise abatement, every home had to be redone with double insulation, new doors, new windows, central air conditioning, new heating; and, our rent hasn't gone up in the last 10 years that we have been living here. Can't beat that with a stick or a poke. And we don't hear the airplanes flying by hardly at all. It's almost quiet as a mouse. And our rent is low and manageable.

I am 82 now and who knows how long I will live. Only time will tell. And it doesn't bother me at all. I don't have a fear of death. God will take care of my family and me as he as always has done in the past.

The last part of the Nicotine Anonymous 3rd Step Prayer says it all:

> Through trust in our Higher Power, we found that we were taken care of in surprising and simple ways. This gave us new confidence and increasing faith. Our victory over our own difficulties encouraged us to continue, and we became an example for others as well.

I quit looking for those Red Sea type miracles. If you keep doing that you will not see the tiny daily ones that we need. Like getting a $10 refund check in the mail or someone bringing you dinner for the evening. Being thankful for all things and thanking Him for what he does. And when I get antsy, and I do at times, I stop and repeat the serenity prayer a few times and ask God to get me focused one more time on where I should be. The times I go through difficulties I experience how God gets me through it then I can be more assured He is in control of my life and knows what is going to happen and He will take care of it. That gives me the encouragement to keep on going no matter what happens.

I am a happy camper these days, and the thing I used to think were important don't mean diddly squat any more. I used to obsess over material things — a new car every year and always the newest gizmo that keeps coming out all the time. Not to mention going on vacations, cruises and all that fun stuff which I don't regret.

The bigger regret would of not having gone anywhere in your life span and have no memories. So I am glad for that.

I still have hope that we might be able to somehow, and I don't how, but to travel all over the US, Canada by car. I would have to win the lotto to do that. But dreams are what keeps one alive. If you have no dreams, that would be sad.

This Program and its 12 Steps for living have been a huge blessing for me, and that is the greatest gift of all. Learning how to live without smoking. I do this one day at a time, and I practice daily living all the time. It's the only way, and without God helping me, I would be a worry wart, angry, fearful, and cynical, you name it I would be it, and I smoked 3-4 hours a day. What a waste of time that was. Smoking and getting these pipe dreams of how to solve my entire problem and I called it meditation… what a joke! Nothing ever came out of those pipe dreams, but I kept on persisting in doing just that.

Now I don't think of smoking anymore, and it's been a good 22 years since I have thought of a smoke. That's a miracle in itself. My biggest fear was how I was supposed to function in life without a cigarette. In fact, it terrified me. Smoking is not an issue with me anymore as long as I live these principles in my life one day at a time. I am an addict, and I always will be. In other words, I am not cured of this addiction. I just don't participate in it any longer just for today. I have no fear of smoking again, but also I will never say I will never smoke again as I do not know that for a certainty. I keep going to meetings, sharing my experience, strength and hope, and being in service. It protects in my new way of life and as long as I do that I will have no fear of returning to smoking. If I say I will never smoke again, then I have signed my death warrant as what I really said is I am cured, and therefore I don't need to come to NicA anymore. Believe me; I have seen this many times over the years.

Smoking was a way of life for me for 49 years and what a waste that was. At the time though, it was my mainstay. I really believed in all my heart that it helped me to be creative, reduce stress in my life, and enjoy life and being happy. Now, all that was a big lie. I was not happy; I hated myself, I just escaped by taking another drag off the cigarette. Life is full of stress on a daily basis. And I found smoking did not get rid of stress, it still remains. I have learned how to deal with stress by looking for solutions and not by smoking and escaping into a dark corner to contemplate how to do what I need to do. It didn't really relax me. All it did was relieve the craving so technically speaking it did relax me for about ten minutes when the next craving hit. I was controlled by that stupid inanimate object called a cigarette. When you think about it that is really disgusting, it's insane, isn't it?

Today I am a walking, talking miracle as I have been given a bonus life of over 22 years. Now that is a pretty neat gift from God. Today on my quit meter it shows I have not smoked 550,500 cigarettes since I quit. Now that is a humongous amount of cigarettes I could have smoked if I could have stayed alive when I was still smoking. That's over a half of a million cigarettes. Or 27,525 packs of cigarettes. And at the price of cigarettes here in California of about five dollars a pack that would be $137,625 dollars not to mention all the doctors and hospital visits, medications, cough syrup, burnt clothing, burnt tables, car seats you name it, and I wouldn't be surprised if that were another $200,000, so the cost of cigarettes really is the least expensive things we purchase to smoke.

But that is all hypothetical as I would have been dead in a couple of weeks anyhow if I didn't quit when I did. There is a good side to smoking though but first, let me tell you the bad part. It kills you! The good part is it takes a long time.

I really enjoy my own company, and that's a blessing. I use to hate myself, and consequently, I hated everyone else. I would point a finger at someone, and there would be 3 pointed back at me and one at God. I can speak my mind and not be threatened by it. I do get a little overbearing at times, but I recognize and try to correct. I used to be so afraid to speak my opinions. Now you can't shut me up.

My makeup, years ago was a person who was very shy especially around women, afraid of my own shadow, a physical coward, afraid of life, a huge people pleaser and a yes man. And the only solution I knew was to smoke. Oh how well I knew to hide behind a cigarette. I am an expert at it. Everything I did had to be pre-empted with a cigarette. I couldn't go to the restroom without lighting a cigarette. I felt I was just taking up space.

Today I am experiencing a new joy of living without all those fears of my earlier years. And for that I am grateful. I am still married for 46 years, and we still get along great, and we still have our nightly silliness. It feels so good to be loved and having someone in my life I can share with and not have to smoke. She hated me smoking and for years made no bones about it.

I don't stink anymore, and my daughter who still smokes visits us and she smells terrible. And to think I didn't stink. Hell, I couldn't smell myself. I thought everyone was crazy. No more yellow fingers, no more hacking or restricted chest pains. I do not miss that one bit.

That was the best thing I have ever done for myself by quitting smoking. My health is a thousand times better, and my spiritual life has improved immensely, and I can stand up for something for a change. That is a good feeling. I love this program, and I am in a lot of services and have been since the day I started quitting. It was not easy, that for sure but being around the support group of my peers made all the difference in the world. It just got easier as the days rolled on. I was hammered with do not smoke no matter what even if your ass falls off. You have to walk through this path of recovery. After all, I am the one who took up smoking and now I had to pay the price of recovery. Sort of like you do the crime you, you do the time. But when you get out on the other side it is so awesome, it unbelievable. And you won't know it till you get there.

Yes, I am grateful, and I show my gratitude by my actions. May it never change.

I'M A NUTCASE

So I'm a nutcase. That's what happens when you're a nicotine addict. While smoking I stayed away from people. I was a mess health wise. I stunk to high heaven, couldn't stop coughing, everyone was on my case about smoking, and my belligerent self told them to go to hell if they didn't like it. I lived in hospitals and doctors' offices on an ongoing basis loaded with meds, cough syrup, cough drops, you name it. And I believed my life was going ok all things considered. After all, I had a right to smoke. As long as I wasn't hurting anyone else, what's the big deal? Of course, I was hurting my family and friends or should I say associates? I really had no friends as I as a loner but as long as I had my cigs, who cared? Basically, I stayed in denial what smoking was doing to me for a very long time.

So now I don't smoke and haven't for many years. I can now act like a nutcase and be glad doing so. At least I am a smober nutcase. And I like it. You know since I quit smoking, my quit meter says I have been able to not smoke 500,500 cigarettes since I quit smoking. My God that is a lot of cigarettes I must say. I smoked up to 4 packs a day and I set my quit meter for smoking 70 cigarettes a day and now I look at the stats, and it's hard to imagine I really could have smoked that many cigarettes if I was still smoking. See what over 22 years of not smoking gets you?

I have been given the gift of smobriety, and it's my responsibility to give it away. As it says in the Bible-"much is given, much is required." The 12th Step states: Having a spiritual awakening as the result of working these steps (the previous 11 steps) we tried to carry this message to nicotine users and to practice these principles in all our affairs. I cannot keep what I have unless I give it away. If I don't I will be like the Dead Sea—always takes and never gives. In which case I would lose what I have gained. It would be all for naught.

So I always share my experience, strength and hope with anyone that comes to mind. I have been through many phases of this addiction and recovery over the years and processing the first 11 steps in my life I practice the 12th Step by helping the newcomer and whoever else comes into my life. The 12th step says to practice these principles in all of my affairs. That means I have to walk the talk in all areas of my life. How one might see me in a NicA meeting, then I best be sure I'm the same way at home, work, or out in the community.

Where I used to think what my purpose in life was, I could not see anything, and I was just taking up space. What I went through by smoking and what I have learned in this program gives me a purpose now. I believe in service work, and over the years I have been involved in many areas, and it has been a joy to do what I have done. It keeps me out of myself and keeps me focused on my recovery.

For me, to stay in service all these years has given me a lot of freedom, and no desire to smoke, none what so ever. Now, this did not come easily to me and to say otherwise would be a lie. This addiction is so buried in denial that after decades of smoking it's almost impossible for one to find a way out of using nicotine.

I smoked for 49 years up to 4 packs a day. I was a basket case, and I spent the last 15 years before I came to NicA on trying quit in any way I could. I could quit, but I couldn't stay quit and that just frustrated me to no end. I have been to countless cessation programs and when they were over with where was I able to go and get support. There wasn't any. I was like on the edge of a cliff and had two choices. Stay nuts with a thought of smoking or smoke. I don't need to tell you what I did. I quit one time and had my own business and my wife send me some balloons and cards congratulating me on quitting and that really irritated me to no end. That put me in a spot of too much pressure to maintain my quit. Needless to say, I went back to smoking. I put my truck two blocks from work and left my cigarettes in the truck, so when I wanted a cigarette, then I walked to the truck. That idea didn't last too long. Ha! That lasted all of one day.

I made my wife responsible for the number of cigarettes I smoked each day. I would buy them and give them to her, and she would give me what I wanted. Each week the amount decreased, and after a time I wasn't giving her any cigarettes to her to dispose to me. I told her this doesn't work and it's a bunch of bull malarkey. I went to church, and the pastor gave me a long talk over how smoking is a sin and all that crap. I took different meds to make me quit supposedly and you know where that went. I have been to hypnotists, therapists, I put myself in the hospital three times due to smoking issues, and that didn't make me quit. A bad case of pleurisy, pneumonia, acute bronchitis, and on and on the list went, and you couldn't scare me into quitting. Hell, I just smoked more to hide the fear. I went to one doctor, and this is a joke. She told me if I didn't quit I would have a massive heart attack with six months. And then she turns around and says if I could just smoke a half a pack a day, it wouldn't harm me. Lol.

ON THE STEPS

Quitting smoking is a major task, and it is the hardest thing one ever had to do. At least it was for me bar none. I am going to talk about inner peace, and that's because I have inner peace and there was a time I did not have that quality. I had utter turmoil. To find this inner peace one needs to start with Step Two:

"Came to believe in a power greater than ourselves could restore us to sanity" In all my actions I did while smoking was insane in all their outcomes. When I was smoking my chest hurt so damn bad, I knew it was going to burst outward in a million pieces and I still had to try and get another lung full of smoke down my lungs. And then cough my fool head off and bitch and moan about why in the hell am I putting myself through this hell and I take another hit and do the same thing. This is insane. Yes, my body is addicted to nicotine was screaming for its hit, and because I was powerless over it, I obeyed every call it made. All God was doing was getting me to the point that I would look toward him to get my sanity restored (of course when did I ever have sanity?) I don't think I ever had sanity, at least not before age 10 when I started smoking.... Lol

"Know, God, Know peace; No god, no peace." After reading that statement tells it all. Without God, in my life, I do not have a chance of recovery from nicotine. God will allow me to smoke as long as I want even unto death. It's my choice. And I almost took it to the outer limits. My pride always said "If there is a way, there is a will" I had no time for God, after all, I can do anything, and if I can't do it, then it wasn't possible to do it In the first place. So who needs God? I didn't. I function quite well without him, at least I am trying to kid myself in utter denial that won't look at the elephant in the living room and if I did see him then all I needed was a bigger room…lol

I came to a meeting when I first came to NicA, and I hurt so bad and couldn't breathe and was dizzy and had to walk up a flight of stairs to get to the meeting room. There was a steel rail, and I just hung over that rail coughing, spitting, gagging and could not breathe, and my chest was so raspy and hurt like hell, and I didn't care if I lived or died, and I wanted another cigarette—now is that insane or what?? I am now 59 years old and smoking four packs a day. I stumbled into the meeting room and my sponsor to be took one look at me and came that close to calling 911 on me. That was my 5th straight meeting, and I quit on my 11th meeting. How I survived those last six days, only God knows.

The 11th meeting I went to was called "The Gratitude meeting" Everyone talked about the gratitude of quitting. I sure the hell wasn't grateful. But that was the day I quit, and that was on Nov 21, 1998, almost 22 and half years. I was like the prodigal son in the pig's sty coming back home to see if his father will take him back. I knew who God was and have known him for a long time, but he just couldn't get me off this smoking crap. I prayed many times to Him just take the pain of quitting away, and I will quit. Well maybe He does do that for some people, but I can tell you that never happened to me. I was giving God a conditional prayer, and He knew it. I started smoking, and He allowed it, and now I had to recover from it and to ask him for the courage to do so. Now I was on the right path. I was fearful of quitting, and I needed the courage to do so one day at a time. I prayed for that courage, and He gave it to me.

As human beings we do have fear and courage is the ability to move forward in spite of the fear, and that courage has to come from God. I had admitted I was powerless over nicotine, and now I had to believe that God could restore me to sanity. That our lives had become unmanageable. I had to correlate that with insanity. So Steps one and two went together except I had become to believe this was too big a job for God, but on the other hand nothing else was working. It was insane to keep doing the things I was always doing, and the results were futile. My insides were tearing me apart from A-Z big-time, and I was losing my life on top of it.

Step Three: Made a decision to turn my life and my will over to the care of God as I understood him.

As a Christian which is my belief I had to start giving God another chance, after all, he has created a lot of miracles in my life except this one, not smoking so I guess I will give Him one more chance. There is a saying in AA that if there are five frogs on a log and one decides to jump off the log, how many frogs are remaining on the log? The answer is five frogs. The frog only made a decision. Now I disagree with this analogy. The right answer to me is four frogs.

Making a decision is an action step. If I make a decision and don't do anything about it, then it means nothing, nada, useless….. I have to follow up that decision with action, and that means praying to God on a daily basis or throughout the day, and asking for the wisdom of what to do and courage to follow through. I am not a robot, and God did give me a free will do as I choose to do. It's up to me to make the right decisions. God wants me in his life, and it's up to me to accept that. My way always led to disaster. My pride would not let me ask for help…unheard of!! But I was at a crossroad—either look upward or die.

Not much choice there was there? And an amazing thing happened, it worked. There are no rules to pray to Him, while driving, while at work, while in bed, while on your knees. So you ask yourself "Well I don't want everyone to hear me praying to God. So who is going to hear you? Only God is. Ha-ha. What are you going to do? Invite an audience. Like I said I am not a robot. I don't need to ask how to drive, how to feed myself, how to dress or anything like that, I already know. It's things that I do not know what to do is where I need help. Like how do I quit smoking and stay like that and hopefully enjoy being a nonsmoker? This is a daily practice for me for the most part. Once in a while being a "self-made man," I think I can handle it, I give God the day off, and in macro seconds I have destroyed the world…lol. It sure doesn't take long.

Step Four: Made a searching and fearless moral inventory of ourselves.

After getting my one year chip I was losing my obsession to smoke, and that was feeling good, but I knew deep inside in order to keep it I had to start working the other steps. I got started on my 4th Step. It wasn't that I was afraid of doing it as I wasn't. It just seemed like so much work to do, and I already had lots of "stuff" going on in my life as it is, but I started on it. I used the AA style of doing the 4th step. NicA has the same style but it's a little different, so it's not copying them. I listed all my angers, hurts, sex problems and other things that were going on that had me on an ongoing rush to hit the oncoming train head on. Who I'm angry with, why was I angry, what was it about, and what part did I play in it. Now, this is a moral inventory. I listed my good points also. An inventory is all you have good and bad so you can see what you want to keep, get rid of or fix. You have to know before you can repair yourself. Things that used to plague me came out as answers as to why I was thinking what I was thinking. This became revelations to me. This was an important step for me as it began to show me who I was, not what I thought I was or who I was showing the world who I was but who I really was, "The Good, The Bad and The Ugly"—the true me.

Step Five: Admitted to God and to another human being the exact nature of my **wrongs.**

Now, this is a humble step to take. It's easy to tell God as you can't see him and it's like talking into the air but to face another human being, well that is another horse of another color. It talks back to you and looks at you as you speak. It is important to share your thoughts with someone you can truly trust. It does not have to be your sponsor. It just has to be another human being. For me, it was three people, my wife, my therapist, and my sponsor. The important thing is to do it. After reading what I wrote to these individuals at first, I felt squeamish as hell, and now I wish I never said anything, but the next morning waking up I felt much freer as I had no secrets left to hide or have to lie. I began to feel I could look you in the eyes and be me. That was a first for me. I always liked the words of this ditty "Everyone hates me, nobody likes me, and I'm going to eat some worms........." Freedom for me was beginning. I was feeling alive and beginning to like me.

Step Six: Were entirely ready to have God remove all the **defects** of character.

Step Seven Humbly asked him to remove our **shortcomings**.

Bill W mentioned some time ago that he didn't't like using the same word in each step.

So in Step 5..." it was the exact nature of our wrongs," Step six "Were entirely ready to have God remove these defects of character" and Step 7 "Humbly ask him to remove our shortcomings."

At first glance, I thought this sounds dumb, all three steps meaning the same thing. What's the point of doing that? One step should solve the problem. But Bill W was right. Here is the deal. Step Five we tell someone our wrongs to another human being as the exact nature of our wrongs, Step Six "Were entirely ready to have God remove all these defects of character" And in Step Seven "We humbly ask him to remove our shortcomings. So we have "exact nature of our wrongs, character defects and last but least shortcomings. All are meaning the same thing but there is a different action to be taken in these three steps. Step five—we tell someone, Step Six—we become willing and Step Seven—we ask Him.

My character defects ran the gauntlet. I lie, I am selfish, false pride, I cheat, etc. and my shortcomings is procrastination, laziness, looking for the easy way out, etc. But in either case, I asked God to take these out of my life, and he did. But the important thing to remember He did take these away from me contingent on my spiritual condition just for today. When tomorrow comes, we start all over again. The Bible says "Today is sufficient onto thee." This is a today only program. Every day I pray for people, myself and ask for things, thy will not mine be done." Use me in spite of my defects. And he does.

Step Eight: Made a list of all persons we had harmed and became willing to make amends to them all.

A lot of this list can come from my 4th step. This is just a list and a list only so someone comes to mind you have hurt put it on the list. All is required here is to make a list and become willing to make amends. It doesn't mean you will make the amend, just be willing to do so.

Step Nine: Made direct amends to such people wherever possible except when to do so would injure them or others.

This step was the hardest step for me. But it was a necessary step to do. If I wanted to stay free from resentments and worry I had to make my amends using my list. It's so easy to blame others, so you get resentment from it. Even if your only 10% wrong that is what you concentrate on making your amend. You are to clean up your side of the street only. Sometimes it's just a matter of facing them and admitting your wrongs in what happened, and others you have to back up what you're saying by proof, like paying a back bill long overdue. Each time I made an amend I got more freedom and less fearful of the world around me.

There are amends you can't make as the people have died or you have no idea where they are. In those cases, you just try not to make the same mistakes, and if you run into someone down the road, well make your amend while you have the chance. And there are times making your amend will hurt someone. You do not have the right to do so just to relieve your guilt like having an affair and telling your spouse about it. My opinion is not to say anything about it and make it a promise to yourself not to do it again. Now others will say pray about it, and I agree to pray about it, but go ahead and fess up...I think that will cause more havoc, but it's up to each person how to handle these type of problems. The important thing to do is to clean your side of the street and not the other person's side. That is a big no-no.

Step Ten: Continue to take personal inventory and when we were wrong promptly admitted it.

My 4th inventory was past issues and Step Ten is a present issue— today. Sometimes I lie in bed and think of what transpired during the day and how I could have done it better. If I have done something wrong I need to promptly admit it and take care of any damage it may have caused. Sometimes I reflect during the day of a conversation I might have had with my wife, friend, customer and something I said was out of place so when I have a chance I give them a call and apologize. I used to think promptly meant whenever I get around to it, maybe in a week or two. The Bible says; "Don't let the sun go down on your anger." That means today or ASAP. As you can see this is a program of daily action.

Step Eleven: Sought through prayer and meditation to improve our conscience contact with God as we understood Him, praying only for knowledge of his will and the power to carry that out.

I have already have a conscience contact with God in Step Three, Five, Six and Seven. Now, this step is to improve the conscience contact that I have. This where we do not find God as we have already discovered him starting Step Two. We are here to improve what we already know. This is where we learn to meditate and ask Him for knowledge of his will for us and the power to carry it out. How does one meditate? Everyone has their way of doing so. Now myself I like to lay still and be quiet and listen for his guidance. The Bible says; "Be still and know that I am God" I learn to shut my head down and just be quiet without any outside influences. Sometimes I am driving along the beach or see a full moon, and it really makes me conscious of who created all of this for us to enjoy. Does God speak to me directly? No. But as I read something, something jumps out at me or maybe through another person like in a meeting one will share something that will stick like a light bulb moment. Or just a thought would pass through my mind. God works in all kinds of ways. I have gotten real neat thoughts while watching a movie.

What's His will for me? Basically to do the right thing. Follow the Ten Commandments. I know what's right and what's not right. Be kind to my fellow man and sometimes that's tough, ha-ha but nevertheless practice that. I try to smile when I am out and about at people that I don't know, and I get a smile back, and I feel good. Being in a long line at a cashier lane can be trying at times. I try to concentrate on reading something or start up a conversation with someone. Then sometimes I just tell myself, "the world isn't going to come to an end if I don't get out of this traffic lane in ten minutes instead of five minutes. This step is where you get to practice the things you have learned.

Step Twelve: Having had a spiritual awakening as a result of working these steps, we tried to carry this message to nicotine addicts and to practice these principles in all of our affairs.

I have gotten a spiritual awakening as a result of working the previous 11 steps, and the 12 Step says to carry this message to nicotine addicts. What message is this? The message of the previous 11 Steps and I work the 12th step by carrying the message. And then I have to practice these principles in all of my affairs. I have to walk the way I talk. Period!! If I don't do that, then I am not working the 12 Step. I am only working 11 steps, and you can't keep it unless you give it away. Guess what happens if you don't give it away? You lose it and all that work for nothing. I become the Dead Sea as the Dead Sea always takes but never gives. I am an addict, and I always will be one, but I am a non-using addict as long as I don't pick up. Being an addict, I always run the risk of using again. If I forget where I came from and didn't give it away, I will lose it. I share my ESH and am very service oriented, and I love it. This program has saved my life I am very grateful for that fact. I have no fear of smoking again; now notice I did not say I would never smoke again. I just have no fear today of smoking again. If I ever say I will never smoke again, then I have just signed my death warrant as I don't need this program anymore and I am gone and outta here. I feel safe today and today is all I need for a nicotine free life. I haven't thought of smoking for a good 21 years now. Now that is a miracle. From a person who would have been dead within a month on the outside, I am alive and well after 22 and half years and plan on living for a few more years.

Through these steps, I have found inner peace with myself, with others and God. I can accept life on life's terms. When I first got here, I was a raving lunatic. I used to kick in doors, throw coffee cups at the wall, break windows, kick my car door, cuss and rant and feel like I am the victim here and now I'm a peace loving person who is not afraid to stand up for something when needed. I don't have all that rage I lived with for years. All I was doing with that rage was hiding my fear, and I was smoking to cover that up, and in the process, I was killing myself. Being free, feels so good in my life today.

THOUGHTS ABOUT STRESS

I want to share my thoughts about stress. My whole life was full of stress from the time I got up until I went to bed. I smoked to relieve that stress. It helped to a degree, but I suspect more so in relieving the craving of a cigarette than the stress, so naturally, I felt better. Each hit of nicotine I used was short lived, maybe 20 seconds and I needed another one. That's why I was smoking up to 4 packs a day when I quit.

I felt better, but the problem I was facing wasn't being taken care of as I just smoked it away. Now stress in itself is a good thing. Every day has stress; it's a matter of how I manage it. And I have to do it without smoking. Stress gets us motivated to do things that need to be done, fixed, paid, work, etc. Without that underlying push (stress) we would just sit on our butts an do nothing, and that causes procrastination, and that leads to stress and fear which leads to resentments. It's an unending battle LOL

So what's the solution? Do the next indicated thing and when it's finished, do the next thing. Try and not to put much thought behind it as it's too hard to do, etc. Just do it, it doesn't feel good, but when you're finished with that chore or confrontation or whatever it is, the feel goods come. I have always felt like I have accomplished something. When I am stuck with a problem or what to say, I ask God to give me the courage to finish what I need to do or put words into my mouth to say what needs to be said.

I find in my life that a good portion of the stress I go through is my own doing. I can eliminate a lot of it by taking responsibly for it. Let's say I see a bald tire on my car, rather than wait until I have a blow out; I buy another tire. That saves one problem I won't have to deal with for a while. Sometimes after work I am really tired, and I need to go to the store, and I am in no mood for it, or I have to get some gas. I will do it tomorrow but tomorrow has a lot of things I need to do. I am not willing to do it tomorrow, so I go to the store and get gassed up and any other things I need to do before I get home. Sometimes it's a little bit of anxiety doing so but when I get home I am greatly relieved, and it turns out to be the best thing I could do to help me out.

I have to help myself out in these areas as they cause me the most problems I have to deal with rather than solve them. I solve one problem, and there is always another one behind it to solve. A thing to learn is to get into the solution and stay in the day. So what does getting into the solution mean? Regardless of the problem, first of all, does it need to be done today? I have enough things to do today than to be bothered by things that can be taken care of next week for example. I can think of some vague ideas but put it aside for the moment and take care of what I need to do today. I look at all the options and then make a decision and go for it. If that doesn't work, try something different. It's not doing anything that gets me into problems. I have to be in control of the problem with God's help not buried with the problem and ignoring it thinking it will somehow magically go away all on its own. All that does is paralyzed me into inactivity and then I blame everyone for my problems. I become my own victim.

I try each night to get a good 7-8 hours' sleep no matter what time I go to bed or when I get up. My sleeping cycle is erratic. I go to bed sometimes 2-4 am in the morning, and therefore I wake up at 11 am to noon time. I worked hard at changing my sleep habits. I go to bed now at 10:30-11:00 pm and get up at 7:00 am. This action gives me a full day to do things. Recognize that stress is part of our life. It's all in how we handle it. Sometimes there is nothing to do about it, and it becomes a fact. I have to accept my outside circumstances as I have no control over most of them.

I recognize that stress not taken care of leads to resentments and that can get you overly worried and make you tired and no energy and in a given time if it's not taken care of in a positive manner, it can lead you back to smoking.

I have found out too that most stress things one has to deal with do not have deadlines even when dealing with creditors or lawyers etc.

I live on a fixed income and my wife always told me to pay the rent first and then we will worry about the other bills. We have to keep a roof over our heads. Of course, I didn't listen to her, and I always paid all my insurance, utilities, etc. first, and there wasn't enough money for rent, and then I would sweat BB'S

Finally, I listened to her and had in the last few years paying the rent right off the top and what a difference that makes.

We would be driving ourselves somewhere and I get lost to a degree, and my wife would say, stop at the gas station and get directions. No, hon, I think I know where I am at, and I just bury myself in deeper because my pride won't let me admit defeat. Now I don't waste any time getting direction if I get lost. Sure saves on the anxieties….ha-ha you live and learn. These are just a few thoughts on the subject. Hope it helps.

Now that you have quit smoking your stress factor does go up by at least ten times as I always buried my pressure points. I made quitting smoking the highest priority in my life. So I just put things on the shelves and did the simple things first and do as much as I can handle. Like I said, nine out of ten times there is no such thing as a deadline.

A funny thought just came to me. I put myself into the hospital as I thought I was having a heart attack, but it turned out to be pleurisy which is very painful in itself. I was in the hospital for five days, and I was wacky as a loose cannon. I drove all the nurses nuts, embarrassed my wife for all my actions I would do things like folding up a lunch menu into an airplane and flipping it to the nurse. I grumbled, refuse to take my pills and just made myself a general pain in the rear. They were glad to see me go. Now that was about 25 years ago. It just occurred to me my actions were due to nicotine withdrawal. It took 25 years to figure that out…..a slow learner ha ha ha

Hope what I wrote helps somebody. Hang in there for another day and each day is different. Nothing stays the same. It will get better, trust me.

EVERY DAY IS DIFFERENT

This has been a weird night. Sometimes nighttime leaves me somewhat unsettled. It's a childhood thing. My dad was an alcoholic, and he suffered from DT's and was always wandering around at night with a baseball bat and breaking things or shooting his gun at rabbits walking on the wall and stuff like that. I always hid in my bedroom under my blankets reading my comic books. It was a safe place for me in those days. And every so often I feel this weird feeling late at nights. It only happens once in a while.

Now that would be nice to smoke over wouldn't it? I don't care how old you are, we all have old tapes that play in our heads. They like to pop out and play havoc with your day. Well, the good side is when it's gone you have a good day, and you really like it. Makes for a good comparison. Thank God every day is different. The staying in the day is so important to me as I live each day. Some days are better than others and that all depends on my attitude for that day. I am really responsible for how my day goes as far as my outlook is on it. Circumstances do not change, but my attitude toward them do.

My wife and I went out for dinner, and on the way home I was in the left hand turn lane and the signal changed and there were three bikers behind me. Two passed me on the right and made a U turn in front of me as I was moving forward, and the other made a U turn passing me on the left. I almost creamed that sucker from one end of the earth to the other. What a bunch of idiots. I wish they would outlaw bikes. I think there too dangerous. I never see them, as there always in a blind spot.

I got over it after I got home….nothing happened so why waste energy on them idiots. Now that would be a good reason to smoke…ha-ha No way Jose. There is always something in my life each day that always prompted me to smoke, but smoking is not an option for me anymore. I go through life each day, and it never occurs to me to smoke. That is a fantastic feeling. This was a weird day as the day went on.

I took my wife to the doctor and forgot my wallet and cell phone, missed turn offs and had to go out of my way to get there and the same thing happened on the way home. We had to pay for parking, and it would cost us a dollar after the ticket was validated. I didn't have a dime on me, and my wife had 60 cents. One of the nurses in the office gave us 50 cents. That was nice of her. So we didn't get locked up in the civil courts. Lol

Stuff like that happens all the time and you have to flow with it, or it will drive you bonkers. So overall my day went well. This is Monday night, and I might get this letter finished tonight or tomorrow. Only the Shadow Knows. I'm very philosophical today…ha-ha. I am 82 and enjoying life to the fullest. Most of my days are pretty good with a bad one thrown in for the hell of it. It makes me appreciate the good days more. And when I look back at my bad days, it was my attitude that sucked and God wasn't in the picture.

GOOD THINGS ABOUT NICOTINE

Now here is something I wrote up about the good things about smoking… LOL

You get to meet new people. Doctors, pharmacists, nurses, surgeons, morticians, religious leaders, and the list goes on.

You can get extended vacations in hospitals at different intervals being able to watch TV. Resting in bed while getting high with oxygen being fed to you or maybe some drug like morphine to relieve some pain you're having, or some tube down your throat to help you breathe easier.

You get to be an expert on a different nebulizer and different medications to see the effect they have on you. You know like chest pains and breathing difficulties…

Sometimes you can take time off work due to smoking, and that gives you a chance to rest up while you crawl on the floor trying to breathe or just doing the jump dance of coughing spasms.

And you don't have to worry about putting money aside as you don't have any in the first place---because it's always going up in smoke.

And you don't have to worry about breathing foul odors as you can't smell anything any way.

And look at all the advice you get from friends, spouses, co-workers, and doctors on how to make your life better. Not to mention about all the sins you can rid yourself of that is brought up by well-intentioned friends and associates.

You learn all about guilt, remorse and total humiliation that you can only learn from by using nicotine. Wow!

Hell, you won't even have to deal with people, they will shun you. That gives you more peace and quiet.

You get to practice hiding in your smoke world where no one can bother you...isn't that great?

And you know what the best part of this whole deal is? Yep!

You get to DIE!

THOUGHTS FROM A JOURNAL

I have recommended new members to start a journal of their feelings for a while to see how things are going. I am enclosing a copy of some of my early journals I still have. Most of them I have lost over the years, but you can get a grasp at how hard it is to stay quit without taking this addiction very seriously.

These are some thoughts I have written in a journal after the first 90 days or so.

Day: 87:

Yesterday was the 1st day I didn't want to go to a meeting (been going 90 and 90). I was tired and kind of bored at the meeting. I woke up this morning feeling the same way. Screw it! It was getting to be a hassle. I called Matt (my sponsor) today and asked him about it. He said you are off your honeymoon trip. Boy did I identify with that. I am going to a meeting tonight, and now I want to go. Now I realize I have to go to meetings to protect myself from not smoking. The responsibility lies with me. I don't have to go to 7 days a week anymore. I do have another life beside Nicotine Anonymous. I am going to try five nights for awhile

Day 100:

I was feeling angry and feeling sorry for myself. I was complaining to my wife about the kids always pulling on us. Telling my wife we never do anything, and she blames it on the meeting—BS! Been that way for a long time. Angry with my daughter, because she doesn't feel we spent enough money on her wedding—screw her! I woke up this morning feeling the same way—wanting a cigarette. I could see it is just an escape mechanism. I guess my feeling is about not having any security when we get older. Called Matt and left a message.

Day 116

Don't want to work—this attitude has to stop, it ruins my day, and then I feel sorry for me, and then I get the urge to smoke. This has been going on for a while. The thought of not smoking has been leaving off and on, and now the real life is seeing some hope. I should be grateful. I guess I am, but I don't know my true feelings. I am going to a NicA panel at a hospital tonight, and I feel kind of phony. I guess I am supposed to be up all the time---expectations too high—that's part of the process.

Day 117

Today is a lot better—Went to a panel last night at Mission Viejo Hospital. Molly, my daughter, is going into surgery for her back at 6 am, and she is going to be in a lot of pain for a while. We will have Andrew, our grandson, for the next 2-3 months until she recovers. Three more days and it will be four months without a cig. That's a miracle.

Day 136

Been going nuts with my emotions lately. I am not sure what I am feeling. Angry at everything, but I can't place what I am angry about or is something I am afraid of? I don't want to be at work, too much conflict with my partner. All we do is fight.

I don't want to be at a meeting—nothing is making me happy

Day 137

I think I finally figured this anger shit out. All the emotions I am feeling now are emotions I've always had but never dealt with them. I smoked them away. The nicotine deadened the anger and fears and was able to hide behind the smoke. So what it amounts to, is that I need to write and talk this stuff thru until it levels out. That is 49 years' worth of smoking and its feelings. How can I expect it to go away overnight? Once the honeymoon was over, it's over. Welcome to the real world! No wonder it's a bitch to stay quit.

Day 138

I got over the physical cravings, but as life goes on, I am fighting these damn thoughts of smoking. Now I have to deal with everything that makes me want to smoke, a phone call, coffee, being hungry, tiredness, anxiety, stress and every conceivable trigger that brings on the urge to smoke. While I am doing this, I have to live and sort out all my emotional garbage.

No way could I do this on will power—it's too weak. I need God's power. It's a miracle for me at 138 days without a cigarette and functioning pretty well, all things considered.

Day 139

My ego is in the way. What I wrote about yesterday has gone to my head. My head is making speeches—oh wise one I am.

So I think of smoking to humble me............sick

Day 143—Tuesday

Much better today—Sat. and Sun. was a bitch. It was fine until Sat. Noon. We were going out shopping for a bike for our grandson for his birthday, and go for lunch. It was getting late, and I didn't want to be late for my meeting. I asked my wife if she was ready, and she said "What's your problem? Think you will be late for your frigging meeting?" And I said yes, and the shit hit the fan. She told me she is hurt and angry because all I can think of is them damn meetings, and I looked at her and thought to myself...*Now what? I didn't have a clue. She has been on my case for smoking for a long, long time and now she is resenting me and the meetings....who can figure?* I tried to talk it out, but I didn't understand why she was feeling the way she was, so we left, got the bike, went home and I went to a meeting.

After the meeting, I was feeling ok. I came out of the meeting, got into my truck and my battery was dead. Shit!

I called AAA and was taken to a station to get it charged. The battery was no good and had to get another one... So while I was waiting, an employee was talking to me with a cigarette waving all over the place, and I was feeling very uncomfortable.

I walked away wanting a cigarette, and went and had a beer (I quit drinking after I quit smoking), and that made the impulse too smoke even stronger. Hanging around the smoker made it worse, so I went and had another beer. I was very hungry, came back to my truck, read my NicA book, and finally, the truck was ready. I drove home really wanting a cigarette.

I thought to myself; *I am not going to make it as a non-smoker regardless how hard I try.* I got home, called my sponsor, and left a message. My wife and I tried to talk lightly for a while, and I went to bed. Matt then called me; we talked for a while. And I felt better. We talked about H.A.L.T (hungry, angry, lonely, and tired). The two things that were bothering me were that I was angry and hungry, plus the fact I was hanging around a smoker. I didn't mention about the drinking—that was my dark secret).

And he told me I should have just gone for a long walk. Two to 3 times on Sunday, my wife mentioned about me being on time for John's birthday. I didn't respond to it. We went to his birthday, and I was angry. I really didn't want to talk to anyone.

We left and stopped for dinner. We tried to talk this shit out, and at this point, I still didn't know what the hell the problem was. I am a time person, and my wife isn't. So why is she pissed at me? I abruptly got up, went outside, counted to 10, came back in and said, "Why don't we just separate for about 6 years, and then get back together when we get our act together?"

We went home, and all I could think of was running. It was too overwhelming—my usual pattern when things get touchy between us.

I wanted to get drunk, smoke myself into oblivion, and go to the casino where I can block everything out. So I say to myself, *what the hell have I learned thru all of this?* Not a thing. I thought God saved me from making a fatal mistake, but I guess not. I remember a member by the name of Chris saying over and over at meetings. "Don't smoke no matter what." Call your sponsor or somebody. I went to bed and called him in the morning. I talked to my sponsor, and after I threw out everything emotionally, he asked me, "What is primarily bothering you?" I said my marriage was on the blink. He told me to make a date and talk this out. "This is killing you, this rage. These intense, sensitive feelings have to go."

So my wife and I talked on the phone, and when I got home, we talked. It turned into a petty argument and got out of hand, as usual. My anger she saw as weakness. My anger was pushing buttons within her that reminded her of her father who physically and sexually abused her all the time.

I have been off and on with my meds. They did calm me down a bit, but I need to stay on them so I can work on myself.

What is the point of all this? To show how intense this crap can really be, and if I don't change, I will remain in my addiction. I had one hell of an anger problem mixed with my drinking, and it was driving me bonkers. I was at a turning point here, and I knew I could not smoke. If I smoked, I would die. I made an absolute for myself, "Smoking is not an option for me."

I had to be willing to go to any lengths not to smoke. I started going to therapy, working the Steps, getting involved in service, and doing a lot of writing. I had to know who I was.

Day 145

Talked to my sponsor today wondering what in the hell is happening to me? I have to go to meetings, and I don't want to. I don't want to go to the conference in Costa Mesa, but I will go. This whole thing is getting tiresome. My sponsor reminded me to think about where I came from, and where I am now. I am being ungrateful. He said everyone goes through it, but we don't dwell on it.

I know my attitude for gratitude stinks, but I didn't believe that was my problem.

Day 147

It's the second day at the conference, and I feel good. I woke up in the morning in the hotel, and I wanted a cigarette real bad. I haven't been in a hotel room by myself since I quit, and that is what I did when I checked into a hotel.….I smoked.

So I woke up, and bingo I wanted a cigarette…*damn this shit is hard, is it really worth it?*

I spent the day at the conference going to marathon meetings. This helped me in my gratitude issues. This will keep me enjoying not smoking. Went to meetings from 10 am till midnight.

Day 150

I feel fantastic—tired but good. It's 6:15 pm, and I'm going to meeting in Costa Mesa. When I am at the meetings, I feel great. When I leave and get home, I want to share with my wife, but I can't. It's like we're in two different worlds. Maybe this is normal with my wife being a non-smoker.

Gary M.

Day 171

Got to work on my anger. It's going to destroy relationships. My partner is getting mad. I come to work with a shitty attitude, and it's getting me nowhere. Sonny and I talked it out. Hopefully, it will improve. I am saying it's because of me quitting smoking, but so is my partner. He contains his anger better. I can get violent very quickly. Well praise God I am not smoking

Day 179

The last 2-3 days I've wanted a cigarette or something that would satisfy me. I reached into my pocket for a mint and said, "Oh shit, where are my cigarettes?" Right out of the clear blue sky.

I've been angry for a while, mainly about my wife's mother and my partner. During that time I didn't really think of a cigarette, but now I am calmed down, and I need something. It's like the anger satisfied me. And now I need a replacement.

Seven Months and 15 days

Yesterday I wanted a cigarette. It's been about two months or so since I really wanted one. But I also know I can't smoke one.

I contribute that to the fact I go to a lot of meetings, and I'm involved with Nicotine Anonymous. I left a message with my sponsor. And I feel better. Since March we have been babysitting 1-5 kids on a daily basis. My daughter bought a condo but waited until the last moment to move. We had her stuff at home, at the shop, at my wife's mother's condo. Both my wife and I have been wrung out emotionally, but in spite of everything, I feel good about not smoking. I never thought that day would get here.

Seven Months and 24 days

I don't want to be at work anymore. It's not fun, and there is always some kind of confrontation with my partner.

I wish I could think of some way of getting out and still make a decent living…dream on Gary. I am grateful I don't smoke, doesn't mean I don't think of one. Right now I think that's a normal feeling. Part of the process. I love Nicotine Anonymous and the people there. It gives me a purpose in life.

Eight Months and 25 days

Friday Evening and ready to leave work and go to a meeting. My partner and I are getting along a lot better now. Hope it stays that way. I am grateful I am not smoking. That's not to say I don't have desires. There just a mild nagging, like missing an old friend. The desires are God's business. I am learning to balance out my meetings.

I gave up the treasurer position on Tuesday nights. This gives me the option of going or not going as I get home too late on Tuesday night. I am also going to give up Saturday's position of treasurer also. I am Secretary for Monday night and Thursday night, which I like doing and will keep the positions. I am going to leave it like that for a while. I've had a feeling about starting a new meeting in the Mission Viejo or San Clemente area. I don't know. We'll see where the wind blows.

That ends my journals. I had more, but I have lost them somewhere. But I hope someone can get something out of this journey of mine. This goes to show you, that you can stay stopped smoking no matter what happens in your life. You just do it. But you have to want it more than anything else.

Over the next 22 years I have really gotten into the Twelve Steps and into service, which has been a real blessing for me. I joined AA, quit drinking, and now I really know what it means to be happy, joyous and free. I stay in service mainly because it keeps me from returning to my isolated life, and I can't keep it unless I give it away. Doing service gives me a purpose for my life to be able to help suffering nicotine addict, and just the pure joy of doing something for someone.

May you find the miracle I have found.

NRTs

What should we talk about now? How about nicotine replacement therapy (NRT)? I have concluded there is no such thing as "Nicotine Replacement Therapy." That is a buzz word the business world came up with from those who sell these items for a profit. There is gum, patches, lozenges, E-cigs and who knows what else.

I smoked, and I used patches for a short period—27 days—and it helped me get nicotine free. But it wasn't a nicotine replacement therapy. It was just another form of nicotine I could use. Nicotine is still nicotine. I have seen members coming to meetings and saying they are addicted to the nicotine gum. No, they are not. They are addicted to nicotine. They choose to chew it rather than smoke it. That's like saying I am addicted to cigarettes. No, I am not. I am addicted to nicotine. If I suck on lozenges and I say I'm addicted to lozenges, no I'm not, I'm addicted to nicotine. The sooner we fully realize this, the better off we are.

Because there is a lower dosage of nicotine and we're not sucking all the smoke and tar into our lungs, it is better for us by a long shot. But it will still kill us sometime in our lives, might take longer, but as it's a lot less poison, we are putting in our bodies.

The TV commercials crack me up. Try our gum, and it will stop you smoking! And in many cases it does, but it doesn't stop the nicotine addiction. And what you wind up doing many times is chewing more gum to make up for the nicotine you have been used to taking. The public is being a fed a big lie. However, I do believe whatever works, works as long as our goal is to be abstinent.

And when we get off the so called NRT's, we still will go through a physical withdrawal, but not as bad if we had gone cold turkey. Do you know what the main difference between gum and the cigarette? We don't have to light up the gum. We still go through all the physical actions with the gum. Unwrap the package, take out a piece of gum, put it in your mouth, and chew, chew and chew some more, and in time take it out of your mouth, and put in another piece of gum…hmmm.

One still has the hand to mouth fixation problem—nothing changes if nothing changes. We are always looking for a softer easier way.

We're always looking for that magic pill that somehow will make quitting easy, but sorry to say it's not available. If I want to quit smoking, then I have to quit smoking. When I got to NicA, I wanted to find a way of quitting without quitting smoking. What can I say? There wasn't much hope for me in those days…lol.

The trouble with the NRT's is you can be convinced they have helped you as you do stop coughing, you breathe better, You don't stink, chest pains go away, etc. etc. So the mindset is its ok to keep using this drug of nicotine because it keeps me calmed down and it's not hurting me. Wrong! This is a poisonous drug that will kill, only take longer to do so.

I cannot take that attitude; I was uncomfortable using the patches. I wanted to be nicotine free, and the only way was quit using the patches. I used them only to the point of getting used to not smoking and taking the hard edge off the withdrawal symptoms. On the 28th, the day I stopped using the patch, and it took a few days to be truly nicotine free. There was still some minor withdrawal to contend with because the patch does have nicotine in it. I drank a lot of water to help flush out the toxins.

And to just quit smoking doesn't get it either. There are Twelve Steps of recovery, and believe it or not, these Steps will truly set us free from smoking or even desiring one. It's a life changer, where I have learned to depend on God for my smobriety—and I still hate that word…ha-ha. I depended on the cigarette for me to stay level headed, be able to function, etc. But that was a big lie too. I truly thought I could not function without a cigarette for the rest of my life. And that terrified me to no end.

CHAPTER 2

STRENGTH

STEP ONE, TWO, THREE

For me, Step One, "We admitted we were powerless over nicotine—that our lives had become unmanageable," was easy to take. I knew that I was powerless for a long time before I ever got to NicA. I was hooked on those damn cigarettes, but I knew there was no way I could quit. I resolved to myself that I was going down with the count, but I sure had no plans on quitting. I had failed to quit smoking so many times. I resolved to myself I am not going to try again. Too much guilt was riding on my shoulder. So I take the tough talk, "So I die, so what?" I'd have another cigarette, and smoke that fear down too.

So I couldn't stay quit on Step One alone. If I went no further, I would do what I have always done—smoke! So I came to Step Two, which says I am insane. And Step Three says let God take care of my insanity. The short version is I can't; He can, I'll let' em. Which, if you're like me, my pride won't let me entirely let go and let God. There was a part of me that said, "If there is a will, there is a way." I figured I have to take care of the problem myself. Well after 49 years of smoking, the whole damn sky fell on me, I couldn't get up, and I realized I couldn't do anything. At that point, I finally surrendered to the fact I knew diddly-squat about life and quitting smoking.

Step Two: "Came to believe that a power greater than myself could restore us to sanity."

Step Three: "Made a decision to turn our will and lives over to the care of God, as we understood Him."

I had prayed to God for many months for Him to take the desire away, and I will quit smoking. Well, He didn't do that, so I figured it was too big of a job for Him also. It just confirmed to me it was impossible to quit smoking. Well, I relented and gave Him another chance. I just said to Him, "God will you help me quit smoking?" I wasn't making a foxhole prayer—as in the past—but a prayer of desperation and God reached out and helped me.

Was it an overnight success? No way. I had to work for it one day at a time. God gave me the courage to not smoke for that day. In fact, it was living hell those first few days. But it did get better each day, a little bit at a time.

I like that last paragraph in our book after the 3rd step prayer: It says "Through trust in our Higher Power, we found that we were taken care of in surprising and simple ways. This gave us new confidence and in increasing faith. Our victory over our own difficulties encouraged us to continue, and we became an example for others as well."

Many times I found how God presented a simple way for solutions and a way to get through those tough moments. The more time I had, it encouraged me to do it one more day. As I went through tough situations without smoking that stayed with me and when I met another tough situation, I told myself I could do this again. The more times I did that, it became a "habit" not to smoke, even just because it was tough. Life has its tough moments day by day. So, the choice for me was, "Am I going to smoke, or am I going to learn another way to deal with the problems by finding solutions for them?"

Nicotine Anonymous gave me the solution to my smoking problems. I was a dead man walking when I came here. It took what it took for me. I mentioned 3 Steps, but there are nine more to go to follow through. I lived on the first 3 Steps in my first year, and after I got my chip, I went gung-ho with the rest of the Steps. By doing so, I lost the obsession to smoke, and it hasn't returned. I am experiencing more of the freedom of living I never knew it existed. I never thought I would ever lose the desire to smoke, but I am here to tell you, I did. It has been over 21 years since I have had an actual thought of wanting a cigarette. My health has improved immensely. Yes, I have done damage to my body from smoking, and I will pay for it down the line. The important thing is, I have lived an additional 22 years of life rather than maybe a month if I smoked. I am using oxygen at night, and it makes me feel better during the day because I sleep better. I have been in the hospital three times for kidney stones, once for a kidney infection, and did 30 days in a nursing home. I had a TIA stroke, but I am still alive and doing what I want to do. The best part is I do not smoke. My lungs are clear, my heart is in good condition, my cholesterol is down, my lung capacity has increased, and my emphysema is in an arrested state. Yes, I have trouble breathing, especially in a hot, humid area, and I take meds and inhalers. Do you want to guess where I would be if I were smoking? I wouldn't be here that's for sure. I would be buried somewhere, six foot under.

Yes, it is truly worth to quit smoking regardless of what health issues you are facing. It has been truly a walk with me and my God, who I know as Jesus. In November I will have 23 years of nicotine free. I would have never thought in my wildest dreams this would be possible. It shows me that miracles do happen. Not smoking after 49 years—up to 4 packs a day—is a true miracle. I can go anywhere, do anywhere, be anything, and even fail at things and not have to smoke. Smoking in itself is not a problem with me. I just simply do not smoke, and when I wake up in the morning, that is not my first thought or is it ever throughout the day as it goes on. Not smoking has become a habit with me.

Now does that mean I am cured? Heaven forbid! As long as I keep coming to meetings and staying in service with this program, I have no fear of smoking today. Will I smoke tomorrow? I doubt it very, very much, but there is no guarantee that I won't smoke. I always say it's about the same the same chance of winning the lotto 1,000 times in a row. I pay my Nicotine Anonymous Life Insurance policy in advance all the time. I will never be cured from being a nicotine addict as long as I live. But I am a non-using addict who is a nonsmoker. I don't like the word ex-smoker. It sounds dirty to me…lol!

FACING CRISES WITHOUT SMOKING

The New Year is upon us now, and hopefully, we all will have a good one. What we don't want to do is smoke. Oh, that would be a bad thing and would screw up our lives big time. Life always has things we have to tend to, and I guess you can call them crises. I have a choice of either solving the problem I am faced with, or go hide and feel like a victim. If I stay in that mind set long enough, a cigarette just might sound good. Heaven forbid!

I have learned the ability to think, reason and make sound decisions most of the time. Right now I am faced with financial issues. I was working maybe five days a month to supplement my Social Security, but that's not available anymore. I haven't seen a lick of work in three an a half months. I am not physically able to work a part time job, because I can't stand on my feet long. I get out of breath with any physical activity like lifting or anything like that. Once I tried to get a job as a driver, and I was on probation to see how I worked out. Well, there was a lot of lifting boxes to the airport and walking and running from one airport to another. I was out of breath all the time and was lightheaded, and they noted this and had to let me go. I was expecting that, so it wasn't a shock.

I used to escape from all that crap by smoking my brains out. Problems like finances are always there, and it's meant for me to solve them with God's help. I can't do this by my fortitude. It would be too lacking in a short time. I know we all have problems, and we need to search out a solution. Maybe it's emotional baggage we carry and have to work on those issues like anger, pity pots, and loneliness, etc.

I was a victim of my emotions, and the only solution was to smoke a cigarette. One after another, day in and day out, and was the problem fixed? No! It was buried in my gut. For years that's what I did. And then when I quit, oh my God, the shit hit the fan!

Smoking like drinking was only a temporary solution to a permanent problem. I was oblivious to all that was around me. And I was like that for years. The Twelve Steps of this program help me sort out my life and teach new ways of doing things. I had to recognize that the way I was doing things was not working. It never did and it never will. So change was in the air. Either I stop smoking, or I die. It became that simple for me. Life is so much better not smoking, and I never knew it could be so. Nor did I believe it would happen. Just the thought of trying to quit terrified me to no end. How in the hell can I cope without a cigarette for the "rest of my life"?

COPING WITH CONFLICT

"Serenity is not the absence of conflict, but the ability to cope with it."

~AA Grapevine

I will always have conflict in my life until the day I die. It's a part of life. I can pray to God for serenity, and He will give it to me the same way if I pray for patience…lol. I have to experience a new way of life by processing these Twelve Steps, to learn about serenity, or it's called, "Living one day at a time." I have learned over the years to flow with whatever happens and stay in the solution. It's a case of being restored to sanity by processing my life with God's help and following the suggestions that are presented to me.

Step Twelve says "Having had a spiritual awakening as the result of working these steps…" What steps? In the preceding eleven Steps, I received this spiritual awakening which I could call serenity. I can handle situations that use to baffle me to no end. I stay in the day and don't get bent out of shape for the most part. I still have my moments but they are rare. It shows I am human—not perfect—and not graduating, but constantly learning.

In effect, my life is much calmer and more enjoyable. Now, what more can I ask than that? I don't smoke and haven't thought of smoking for a very long time now. It's been at least 21 years since I thought I wanted to smoke. That is a miracle. My life has become so much simpler these days. May I have many more days to live that way! God has been in my recovery since I got here, and I sure as hell couldn't do anything on my own with any fulfilling satisfaction. I thank God every day and hope for a good day.

STEP FIVE, SIX, SEVEN

The one thing I can enjoy is being a non-smoker. Now that is fun. If I was still smoking and living now, I have no idea how I would survive. If it's kind of bad now without smoking, how much worse it would be smoking. Oh yeah!

The last thing I would ever want is a cigarette. If I light up a cigarette, I would have to ask myself, "Do I want to die?" The obvious answer is NO, so I don't entertain thoughts like that. I remember I used to say what the hell, you gotta die of something. Just another form of denial.

At least when I was smoking, I knew where I was all the time. When it all came down to it nicotine was my drug of choice. I smoke, I die. I drink, I get drunk. That was a big difference to me. Nicotine is a mood altering drug, and I liked the feeling that "everything is ok" while smoking. An escape hatch for sure. But as time went on that didn't work anymore. And over a period of time, I finally quit smoking. And just quitting smoking didn't get it for me. I am expert at quitting but a miserable failure at staying quit. When I did quit, I was very desperate to do so. It was that desperation that kept me smober as I was willing to go any length to not pick up, no matter how bad I might have thought that a smoke would be good. This is where the Steps come into play. It's a matter of change, and that for me meant changing everything I thought was good. When it came down to it, in my thinking of what was good and what was bad, I had no clue what was good or bad.

Thinking can make me dangerous. The one thing I can't do in this program is analyze everything that comes about. Just do what is suggested by other members. "Utilize, don't analyze." If everything in my life didn't work to achieve me quitting smoking, then why did I keep on doing the same things over and over again finding out it still doesn't work? That is insanity! And I couldn't really see why I did things the way I did until I started writing about it. Then things came to mind. I could see a pattern forming in my life experiences.

Then you get into Steps 5, 6 and 7. This is where I began to get my sanity restored. I literally had to find out what was insane and what wasn't insane before I could begin to be restored to sanity. Bill W mentioned some time ago that he didn't't like using the same word in each step.

So in Step 5..." it was the exact nature of our wrongs", Step six "Were entirely ready to have God remove these defects of character" and Step 7 "Humbly ask him to remove our shortcomings".

At first glance I thought this sounds dumb, all three steps meaning the same thing. What's the point of doing that? One step should solve the problem. But Bill W was right. Here is the deal. Step Five we tell someone our wrongs to another human being as the exact nature of our wrongs, Step Six "Were entirely ready to have God remove all these defects of character" And in Step Seven "We humbly ask him to remove our shortcomings. So we have "exact nature of our wrongs, character defects and last but least shortcoming. All meaning the same thing but there is a different action to be taken in these three steps. Step five—we tell someone, Step Six—we become willing and Step Seven—we ask Him.

An exact nature of my wrongs might show I am a thief. The character defect would mean to me, a dislike of working for a living and a shortcoming would be not having the fortitude to go out and look for a job. I wanted things handed to me on a silver platter. So I went through life not getting anywhere, because I had too many things going on in my head. I kind of like my thinking on this. Works for me.

STEP SIX

Step Six: "Were entirely ready to have God remove all these defects of character." All this step requires is become willing to have God remove my defects of character. Smoking helped numb these feelings, and I could deceive myself into believing it was working. As I buried all my feelings and inabilities by smoking over the years, the smoking stopped working and feelings kept bubbling out of my mouth. I smoked more to overcome that, and it got worse. All I was doing was killing myself a little bit more each day. Physically I was a wreck and dying in front of everyone.

As I looked over my inventory and 5th step I could see where I was coming from, and I could see what changes I needed to make. I had to learn to be honest with myself. If I was honest with myself, then I didn't have to worry about being cash register honesty. That was a natural step by being honest with myself. A lot of defects were like a two edged sword. In one way they were good, but on the other side of the coin, it harmed me. An example out of our book, *Nicotine Anonymous: The Book,* is being judgmental. If I was judgmental over someone or something, it helped build up my own self esteem, and I was able to accomplished things in my life. But the downside was, I was separated from other people and remained aloof. It really made me feel useless. And friends were few and far between.

I tried to run my life by smoking. And in the beginning it did help, but it turned on me over the years. It was hard to quit smoking, but it wasn't too hard. And not as hard as I thought it might be.

WANTING TO NOT SMOKE MORE THAN SMOKE

For anyone still struggling to stay quit, don't give up. I came to NicA and they really messed up my smoking. There was definitely no peace in smoking anymore. Every time I lit up and started smoking, I could hear other member's voices in my head saying what would happen—I couldn't shut my head off from these voices. I knew I was powerless over nicotine long before I came to NicA. I just told myself, "So what?" because I wanted to smoke. Smoking pleasures overrode the discomforts of smoking for a long time. It's when I was faced with the reality I was dying, and it was in the sweet good bye, and in the very next few days or weeks. I had to get to that place before I could even think about recovery.

There was no way I would even think about working the Steps of this program as long as I wanted to smoke more than not smoke. What for? Why would I want to do that? All I wanted was the pain to go away so I could smoke, which made the Steps stupid to me. I mean after all I still "enjoyed smoking." I am not sure what that meant anymore.

The one thing I did know was that I was tired of quitting and then lighting up again. That was just too hard to do anymore. You know when I got into recovery? When the pain of smoking was greater than the pain of quitting, that was when I looked for a truthful answer in my life. I was sick and tired of being sick and tired of smoking. It held nothing for me. I came to the fact I was powerless over quitting smoking. I was powerless over my ideas of cutting back or controlling my smoking. I was powerless over using my ideas to quit and nothing worked. In the process my life was insane, and all my actions proved that I was insane. I was open to the idea that other member's ideas had promise, and I was willing to let God help me to stay quit. I was told to go to meetings and just not smoke for today only.

So I began to jump into the Steps, went to a lot of meetings and got into service work as the months went by. In the first year it was hard, but got easier as time went by, one day at a time. For me, I didn't really experience true recovery until I did my Fourth Step, and that was after I got my first year chip. I could have done it sooner, but it represented a lot of work for me. I asked myself if it was really necessary. After I almost relapsed in my 11th month, I realized I needed to move forward and do it. It was the best move I ever did. Then I followed with my 5th step, and onward to the next steps. I felt freer from this bondage of smoking as I moved forward into the Steps. It became a part of my life.

I lived the line, "Don't smoke no matter what, even if your ass falls off," and that is a very true statement. There is nothing having a cigarette would do, nor could that help me in any manner. If I smoked, all it would do is kill me. It was a guaranteed death sentence for me. Quitting the use of nicotine is the best thing I have done in my life. I pray, I go to meetings, I stay in service, I share my ESH and I live! A pretty good deal if you ask me.

LIVING WITHOUT SMOKING

I do this one day at a time and I practice this kind of daily living all the time. It's the only way, and without God helping me, I would be a worry wart, angry, fearful, and cynical, you name it I would be it, and I smoked 3-4 packs a day. What a waste of time that was. Smoking and getting these pipe dreams of how to solve my entire problem and I called it meditation— what a joke! Nothing ever came out of those pipe dreams, but I kept on persisting in doing just that.

At one time, smoking was my mainstay. I really believed in all my heart that it helped me to be creative, reduce stress in my life, and enjoy life and being happy. All that was a big lie. I was not happy, I hated myself, I just escaped by taking another drag off the cigarette.

Life is full of stress on a daily basis. And I found smoking did not get rid of stress, it still remains. I have learned how to deal with stress by looking for solutions, and not by smoking and escaping into a dark corner to contemplate how do what I need to do. It didn't really relax me. All it did was relieve the craving. So technically speaking it did relax me for about ten minutes until the next craving hit. I was controlled by that stupid inanimate object called a cigarette.

Today I am a walking, talking miracle. I have been given a bonus life of over 22 years. Now that is a pretty neat gift from God. Today on my quit meter it shows I have not smoked 575.000 cigarettes since I quit. Now that is a humongous amount of cigarettes I could have smoked if I could have stayed alive when I was still smoking. That's over a half a million cigarettes. Or 28,750 packs of cigarettes. And at the price of cigarettes here in CA of about five dollars a pack that would be $201,250 dollars not to mention all the doctors and hospital visits, medications, cough syrup, burnt clothing, burnt tables, car seats you name it and I wouldn't be surprised if that was another $200,000, so the cost of cigarettes really is least expensive things we purchase to smoke.

But that is all hypothetical. I would have been dead in a few weeks anyhow if I didn't quit when I did. There is a good side to smoking but first let me tell you the bad part. It kills you! The good part it takes a long time.

I really enjoy my own company, and that's a blessing. I use to hate myself and consequently I hated everyone else. I would point a finger at someone, and there would be 3 pointed back at me and one at God. I can speak my mind and not be threatened by it. I do get a little overbearing at times, but I recognize and try to correct. I used to be so afraid to speak my opinions. Now you can't shut me up.

Years ago I was a person who was very shy especially around women, afraid of my own shadow, a physical coward, afraid of life, a huge people pleaser and a yes man. And the only solution I knew was to smoke. Oh how well I knew how to hide behind a cigarette. I am expert at it. Everything I did had to be pre-empted with a cigarette. I couldn't go to the restroom without lighting a cigarette. I felt I was just taking up space.

Today I am experiencing a new joy of living without all those fears of my earlier years. And that I am grateful for. I am grateful I am still married for 46 years and we still get along great, and we still have our nightly silliness. It feels so good to be loved and having someone in my life I can share with and not have to smoke. She hated me smoking, and for years made no bones about it.

I don't stink anymore. My daughter who still smokes visits us and she smells terrible. And to think I didn't stink. Hell, I couldn't even smell! And I thought everyone else was crazy. And today, no more yellow fingers, no more hacking or restricted chest pains. I do not miss that one bit.

Quitting smoking was the best thing I have ever done for myself. My health is a thousand times better and my spiritual life has improved immensely. I can stand up for something for a change. That is good feeling.

I love this Program, I am doing a lot of service work and have been since the day I started quitting. It was not easy, but being around the support group of my peers has made all the difference in the world. It just kept getting easier as the days rolled on. I was hammered with "Do not smoke no matter what even if your ass falls off." You have to walk through this path of recovery. After all I am the one who took to smoking and now have to pay the price of recovery. Sort of like "You do the crime you do the time." But when you get out on the other side it is so awesome, it unbelievable. And you won't know it till you get there.

RECOVERY IS HERE IF YOU WANT TO FIGHT FOR IT

In the beginning, I often thought to myself when I was smoking, *this ain't gonna get it but I don't have a choice. I have to smoke; it's the only thing that keeps me going. It's the only thing that makes me want to live. Without my cigarettes, hell, I might as well be dead.*

Now that is sick, let me tell you. But to see myself as a non-smoker was a useless exercise that was never going to become a reality. Yeah, there have been fleeting moments I wondered what it would be like if I didn't smoke, but they were rare and fleeting. So I lit up a cigarette and dispensed with the whole idea.

I played around for 20 years trying to stay quit and nothing worked, so why was I doing this if I wanted to smoke and if everything I did to quit didn't work? Didn't make much sense to me—this was nuts!

I knew I couldn't quit.
I knew life would suck without a cigarette.
I knew I would die with a cigarette.
I knew it would scare the crap out of me to quit.
I knew it was impossible to stay quit.
Why can't I quit when everyone else can?
Why doesn't anyone understand why I can't quit?
Why do I beat myself in the head like I do?
Why does everyone make me feel so frigging guilty?
Why am I like this?

A babbling idiot for sure! When I got here to Nicotine Anonymous, I wasn't sure about anything. After my first meeting, a guy talked to me forever, and all I could think of was wishing he would shut the hell up so I could go have cigarette. He kept on rambling about God and stuff, and I just shut him out and watched the time. Then when I got to my truck, I was feeling so guilty about lighting up, I had to drive a block or two looking out my side mirrors before I lit up. I just knew they were going to check up on me. It was a downhill slide from there. I couldn't defend my smoking anymore. What a revolting situation this turned out to be. I was forced into a life of abstinence from nicotine.

What in the hell did I let myself in for? Somehow I knew deep inside I would have to quit now and not later, that there was no later—this was it.

So after going to ten meetings in a row, bitching and complaining like the idiot I was, I quit on a Saturday in the middle of the afternoon a few days before Thanksgiving. Who can figure that? Not I, says the man I am. And with cigarettes left on me…that's nuts!

I tried quit dates and all that stuff. I finally I resolved myself to an early death, but would keep my faculties about me. That was how I felt when I woke up on the 11th day after my first NicA meeting. Then in the middle of the afternoon, it just happened. I got this overwhelming feeling like why fight this anymore? Does it really make any difference? Just quit and be done with it!

Now that was a light bulb moment. Praise God and hallelujah and all saints be preserved. I am free of smoking. Yeah! I closed my garage and went in the house and put on a patch and turned on the TV and I really felt free from smoking. And one hour later I was a lunatic wanting a cigarette…so much for freedom. Oh my God! What do I do now?

I looked in the meeting directory and there was a meeting at 4 pm, and if I hurried I could get there. It was only 3:15 but it was 35 miles away. Aw hell! So without thinking about it too much, I just went, and now I am like those batteries….just keep on going and going and going.

I got my first day in and really felt good about it even it was only a half a day. So I was lying in bed really feel good about myself and slept very soundly.

I opened my eyes at daylight and first thought was go out to the garage and have my cigs and I thought aw shoot, I quit last night, damn it! Oh, let me tell you that 2nd day was a mother. I went to a meeting that night and someone was talking about sleeping the day away as they couldn't face the idea of facing another day without smoking. And I thought to myself, what a crock that is! It was being wimpish.

So the 3rd day I slept it away...what can I say?

I just kept doing this one day at a time, and it got easier as time went by. It was hard but doable, and the more time I got behind me, gave me hope that I could really quit. The thing that was bothering me was, would I ever lose the desire to smoke? I heard members saying that it will go away by working this program.

Well that gave me some hope, but I kept asking myself if the desire goes away in time why do members with "x" amount of years still come to these damn meetings? Haven't they learned how to lose the desire to smoke? Is this what I have to look forward too? At the same time I was glad to see them around because it meant something does work here. If they hadn't have been here, I would have thought to myself, *you know what? This is bull cocky here, I am outta here.*

I was full of questions and doubts but I kept on coming back and not giving up. One more day, that's all I had to do. An amazing miracle happened to me after a couple of months of smobriety. At the end of the day I looked back and thought to myself, *I haven't really thought about a cigarette today!* I thought that was the most awesome feeling I have had in a long, long time. You talk about hope...it abounded then.

I was noticing something that was kind of scaring me. I noticed the newcomers that were coming in were going back out, and just the old timers stayed and every once in a while a new old-timer joined the old-timer gang. It was a slow growth process here. I had some time behind me and I wanted to stay smober. So I observed what was going on.

If I want to be an old timer then, I better do what the old timers are doing. Go to meetings, get a sponsor, work the Steps, work with newcomers, get into service, and make yourself available.

I had to pay my premiums on my life insurance policy of Nicotine

Gary M.

Anonymous. This insured that I wouldn't smoke for today. And that's all I have, just today. I stopped arguing and started listening and doing. That was the beginning of my growth. And as time went on I lost the obsession to smoke—an impossible dream that came true!

So it is here for you if you want to fight for it. I can attest to that, it is real for me!

CHAPTER 3

HOPE

SHARING YOURSELF

> "We learn first-hand the truth of the saying that we cannot
> fully know our own story until we share it with others."
>
> —Nicotine-Anonymous the Book.

I like to say "You can't really know yourself until you share yourself." This was an important step in learning about myself. As I shared and learned about my own story, I learned why my story came about and what I could do about it.

By sharing about myself, I got out of myself little by little. At first, I thought I would make a mockery of myself, but I found I could speak my mind and by doing so, I could listen to feedback if I wanted to—of course, I didn't want to in the beginning unless the other members agreed with me. Eventually, I started to listen and use what was being said. And lo and behold, things started to get better.

Want to be in the middle of the herd, as it's often said? Then jump in and get your feet wet! No one is going to make fun of you. We all have been there in one form or another. By sharing and listening, it reinforces to me that I am a nicotine addict and I cannot smoke, not one filthy cigarette, even if my ass falls off. It's better if it falls off than light one up and have to start all over again—fight the awful guilt and regret and a loser's attitude. You can glue your ass back on with "Instant Glue" LOL.

If I want to know something I can ask a question, and I will get feedback. I really wanted to know what made me tick. I was sick of being ticked off over this addiction. For me, facing death was like a holiday. I thought anything is better than smoking again. Even dying.

By sharing you help yourself as well as someone else, whoever is listening or reading. I liked listening to newcomers because it made me feel, "Yeah, that's me." Listening to newcomers helps me feel at home among my peers.

In all the years I have been clean, I still get into myself. It's necessary for me to share so I can get out of the ego me. I can get the poor me's, and I will clam up. I am never cured of my emotions, and they can work negatively against me. The daily cure? Talk about them honestly and clear the air. By doing so, you may be helping someone beside yourself. It's a win-win situation.

My Quit date: Nov 21 1998, which was a Saturday at 2:15 pm which, and as of now, computes to 2 years, eight month, I have not smoked 550,000 cigarettes computed at about 70 cigs a day, and I have saved based on about $2 a pack comes to $48,020. Not bad for a stubborn old dude. The only thing that bothers me is where in the hell is all that money?

WHY CAN'T YOU JUST QUIT?

People who never smoked do not have any iota of an idea what it's like to be a nicotine addict. They think we are nuts to keep smoking when we know it's going to kill us. I had a neighbor always telling me I need to quit smoking. Yeah, yeah, shut your mouth. I made the mistake of saying I can't quit, and he asked that unanswerable, "Why can't you?" Just throw them away and be done with it. Not only could I not answer the question I was highly embarrassed about it.

The only thing that helped me was Nicotine Anonymous. It was what I was searching for, for many years. Until then I failed miserably to quit and stay quit. I have my life back, I have my sanity back, and I have my health back. And I have saved all kinds of dollars. And since I have quit, I have not smoked 550,500 cigarettes to date.

And if you line them up, end for end based on 4" each that comes to a cigarette that is 31.3 miles long.

Nice statistics, huh?

No Cool Hand Luke

Oh, those beginning days were horrendous. Anger, you don't even know the meaning of it. I was in a meeting in the beginning days, and I couldn't keep my mouth shut. I was "sharing," and someone cut in on me, and I slammed my fist on table two or three times and told him to shut the f.... up. I got the floor.

I was not Cool Hand Luke in those days. I came home from work, and the kids and my wife were laughing. I just went into the kitchen where they were at and at the top of my voice, I screamed: "Will you all shut the f.... up or else!" All was quiet, and I turned and walked away. I had so much rage within me; I couldn't tell you why or what or how it happened, nor did I care.

After a couple of weeks, I began to realize I can't keep jumping down everyone's throat. Maybe at times, I had a right to be angry, but it was the way I displayed it that was wrong. I came to the conclusion if I want to stay off nicotine, I best become willing to do whatever I have to do not pick up a cigarette.

I gave up on all my smoking friends, and no one was allowed to smoke around me, in my house and especially my truck. I didn't go to a family function during the holidays, because several people smoked. I was rude and didn't care, but I did not want to place myself in harm's way. I knew I was wrong in my actions, but I also knew I could take care of those infractions at a later date. If I smoked, I could not do anything, because I would probably die in front of everyone. It was hammered in my head, "Do not smoke no matter what even if my ass falls off!" And if I died because of smoking, then everything was a moot point.

So I began an effort not to blow up at everything that came in front of me. It's not their fault I can't handle my anger issues so why blame them? I had to look at myself, what I was doing, and work hard at controlling myself.

I went to meetings and learned to listen rather than talk. Then I put into action what I learned to see if it would fit me. Sometimes it did, and other times it didn't. After a few months, I started to get into service, and that was a godsend for me. Service helped me get out of myself. That was 22 years ago. I have come a long way since then. Believe it or not, today there are many times I refuse to get angry. It's not worth the powder to blow it all to hell!

There is nothing wrong with anger; it's how you handle it. You can either go on a killing rage or talk it out. Communications is the key. The Twelve Steps have helped me immensely in seeing who I was, why I was insane, and what I had to do about it.

The acronym HALT says not to get too hungry, too angry, too lonely or too tired. It does not say it's wrong to be hungry, angry, lonely or tired. It say do not get TOO hungry, angry, and lonely or tired. The one thing I have found is to get a good night's sleep no matter what. I am a Dr. Jekyll/Mr. Hyde personality. If I get too tired, I will let you know.

If I am rested, then my day can go smooth as silk. I flow with problems, enjoy the day, and if I get angry over something, then I deal with the anger before the day is over with. I need to talk it out and resolve it, if possible.

Sometimes it can't be resolved, so I accept it, as I did my part. It becomes an objective fact at that point.

It's not worth it to explode over everything. Many times something happens, and I say, "Oh well," onward and forward. I gave up trying to be the fixer. I couldn't fix things then, and I can't fix things now, so why not give up the idea of being a fixer, and just enjoy life for today?

And that is what I do today! And the most important thing is I do not smoke today. That is the good life.

ANGER BASED ON FEAR

Most anger is fear based. I have to search out that fear and resolve it, and the anger dissipates, subsides, or completely goes away.

Being assertive without being aggressive or passive is a good practice too. It can relieve a lot of anxieties. I have learned to pick my battles. If I am going to confront someone that has made me angry, I make a point of sticking to the issue. I don't get side tracked and didn't threaten or curse at them because I will lose the battle. Then, if they are on the defensive, and I meet them again, they're ready to fight. I can't win.

Sometimes it's better to lose the fight if you get what you want. It's not worth the effort to spout off what is bothering me, especially if I find out I'm getting what I want, even though I may not get it my way.

If I can't let go what's bothering me that can be a key anger issue I need to resolve to find peace. Sometimes problems can't be solved; then the problem becomes a fact. I do what I can do, and that's all I can do. And then I let God take over from there and, then go about my business.

BEING PREPARED

This is a sneaky and deceiving addiction. I have been off the cigs for almost two decades, and I have lost the obsession to smoke. I thank God for that.

However, as an addict, there are times when out of the blue, for no known reason, I might reach for a cigarette in my pocket. That is not an obsession nor a thought of smoking. My brain has been wired for over 49 years of smoking, and it has all the memory of those 49 years, so on occasion, some dumb thought hits me like "a cigarette would sure be nice." You don't say?

I have to destroy those thoughts as fast as they come. That doesn't happen every day, just once in a great while. Like when I am enjoying the outside and the wind is gently blowing in my face, and the thought of having one would really go with the mood. Sure it would.

Something triggers my brain, and my brain answers the trigger. Now it's up to me to deal with it. I never fantasize these thoughts, I just reject them for what they are. The addiction is talking.

Maybe once a year I have what I call my annual smoking dream. It doesn't bother me at all anymore. I have no control over what I am dreaming. It wakes me up, and I think, "Oh a smoking dream," and go right back to sleep. Chances are I won't remember it when I wake up, but maybe the next day I do. I have to laugh at that stuff.

I don't smoke no matter what even if my ass falls off. If it does, I pick it up and use super glue to put it back on. LOL. I have super glue on me or in the car for these emergencies. Ha-ha. The good thing about all this stuff is it gently reminds me I am an addict, and I cannot be cured of it. I don't feel guilty about having a smoking dream; it is what it is.

In the 12th Step in our book, it says: "Nonetheless, we remain addicts. And when we begin to experience the joys of being free from using nicotine, we run the risk of thinking once again that we can control things. That is the risk of being an addict. As the suffering of our nicotine past recedes, the temptations that got us in trouble returns. This brings us to the latter parts of the Twelfth Step—the action plan for continuing to live free from nicotine.

We have learned the best way to keep our madness from resuming control of our lives is by sharing our new gift of life with those who are still suffering. We call it "carrying the message." We do this in two ways; we give away the gift we have received through sharing, and we let our lives be examples for others.

For me, the best insurance is never to forget I am an addict and always be available to help someone out. I stay in service, and that keeps me from getting into myself. I was given this gift from this program, and I give it back freely.

If I am coming in front of people who are smoking, I just hold my breath until I am past them. I don't make a habit of hanging around people who smoke, because we have nothing in common, and I don't like smelling that smoke. I feel safe wherever I go. Hell, I can go to liquor stores, supermarkets, drug stores and wherever they sell cigarettes, and I see them on the shelf all the time. It doesn't bother me a bit. It's just something the store is selling, and I am not interested in them. That's a lot of freedom. It's a wonderful life being a non-smoker. I am incredibly grateful.

I don't like the smell of smoke. It's very nauseating and smells like crap. But it's funny. If I happen to be at a certain distance from the smoker, it smells so good and sweet. If I am 2 inches closer or 2 inches further it stinks like hell. I find that funny.

So then my insurance payments for my freedom is, to go to meetings, be in service, and have an attitude of gratitude as a day by day predisposition. I like what it says in our book. "You don't get to know yourself until you share yourself."

That was the best way I could learn about myself. Speak out if you want help. The more that I spoke out, the better I got to feel good about myself. I don't know if that is good or bad, because you can't shut me up sometimes.

Today is a good day.

Gary M.

THE INSANITY

Bronchitis was my middle name. The last nine months of my smoking career was spent with acute bronchitis day after day, and I thought I would never quit coughing. It hurt so much to cough, and I was not able to breathe. I was waiting to break a rib, but happily, I didn't. After work, my wife would not let up on me about my smoking, and I would go in the bedroom and hang onto the back of the bed poster and just jump up and down coughing, coughing, and coughing, and sometimes find myself on the floor. I was also a phlegm machine. It was all over me all the time. Sometimes I would see blood and then smoke more to hide that. How I managed to get through those nine months is beyond me.

I know God had a hand in it, or I wouldn't be here. Every night I swore off the cigarettes—that is it—and went to bed. I laid down on three pillows and cough for maybe 45 minutes before I could go to sleep, and then wake up in the morning and forgot all about my pledge to quit. I did that for 270 days. I lived with backaches and headaches due to coughing. I drove to work and home, coughing my head off. I got really faint and almost blacked out for lack of oxygen, and drove my car like this every day.

I hated what I was doing, but I could not stop. I would get so pissed off, I would throw a pack of cigs out the window, and then immediately drive to the liquor store to get more. I couldn't wait until I got home so I could go out in the garage and smoke myself to oblivion. I had a roll of paper towels, and I used them up every other day. I could not stop the coughing or phlegm or blood or any other color that was floating in my system.

Now, do you think that was insanity? Nah, just a little problem with the wrong brand of cigarette. Those generic cigarettes will get you every time. I got on the kick of buying the ultra-type smokes with the holes in the filter. I didn't like them so I wrapped the filter with masking tape so I can feel it going down me. I did a whole carton like that. That took some doing. That is not insanity. That was experimenting. Oh yes, whatever works, huh?

And to think in the last few years I was smoking 3-4 packs a day and once in a while on a really insane day; I would smoke five packs. I was at a casino with my daughter, and I was pretty drunk, but I smoked a pack in less than 2 hours. I couldn't stop gagging, coughing, spinning around like a top, and I finally had to sit on the floor by the elevator. The security guards were trying to help me; my daughter was scared out of her mind. I just said, leave me alone, I will be okay in a few minutes.

That's not insanity. I just smoked too many beyond my normal range. That's all, I was a fighter in those days...yi yi yi.

I never want to go through that crap again. I quit on Nov 21, 1998, and if I didn't quit when I did, I would not have seen the New Year come in. I was toast, and I was burnt to a crisp. The only fight I'm going to be doing is staying smober. That's where the real fun begins...lol

CRAVINGS

I hear many times, "Does the craving ever go away?" or, "How long do these cravings last?" I smoked for 49 years, so I have 49 years of conditioned responses in my brain. So after I quit, the cravings lingered on for some time. The thing is by staying on target with your quit, the cravings will relent, a little here and a little there, and finally you don't think about them anymore at least for all practical purposes.

Those 49 years of responses are still in my head, and every once in a while I get this tiny nudge. I can't stop those, but I can accept them and let them go. And that's what I do. A gentle reminder I am an addict. I will never be cured, and to tell you the truth, I don't want to be cured for the simple fact that if I am cured, guess what?

I have to stay on target with my recovery, so I don't fall for some idiot thought that might sound good to me. The slogan we have "We are one puff away from a pack a day" is very true. However, I don't worry about it, because I am a long way off from the "puff." By going to meetings, being in service, and applying the principles of this program in my life, then I do not have to worry about the "puff."

Life is super good without smoking, and I am grateful that I quit, and it has been a couple of decades since my last cigarette. And that is a miracle. It's me, God and this program that has and will keep me nicotine free.

CRUSHING TOBACCO

To keep a pack of cigarettes—or even one cigarette—around is playing Russian roulette. I'm putting myself on a suicide watch. To keep one on hand "just in case" is dangerous, because in "case" will inevitably happen, and I have my famous cigarette handy.

When I quit which was on a Saturday, I had a half a pack left. I was out in the garage, and I climbed a ladder and put that pack of smokes as high as I could and buried in a box on the top shelf and stacked everything around it. If I am going to have something on hand when that moment comes, I want to make it as hard as I can to get it. Ha!

One hectic day at my business, after driving 60 miles from work to home, the traffic was heavy as hell, and it was Wednesday, and I wanted a cigarette in the worst way. You know that I knew where one was. Just in case...

I couldn't wait until I got home and drove up into the driveway. I opened the garage, dug out my ladder, got into the box where those cigarettes were, and climbed back down. A big smile was on my face as I looked at my "'friend" and then I walked to the trash can and thought for about two nanoseconds. I crumbled them all up like dust, and down into the trash, it went.

The miracle of this was the thought of smoking went away. No ashtrays, no lighters, I even took the lighters out of my car. No more hidden stashes or paraphernalia on hand "just in case.

WE ARE ADDICTS

When I came into my first NicA meeting, I didn't know what to expect. I really had the feeling this was the last building on the block. That was a strong feeling that stayed with me. I knew if I smoked I would die. As I sat down on the chair at the table, I looked around, and there were different times of being smober. There was one person of 4 years and another of 7 years and one at two months, and some with just days or weeks.

I was glad to see this amount of time, but when I thought of someone having four and another seven years, I asked myself, "Why are they still coming if they have quit and not have any thoughts of smoking?" Maybe they have been brainwashed. I didn't know, and that bothered me. On the other hand, if I didn't see real long time free of nicotine here, I would leave as there is no proof it works. It took me a while to figure out this difference.

We are addicts, and we will always be addicts, and we will never be cured. I have to come to meetings, so I'm reminded of that fact. As it says in our promises, "We begin to forget we had been nicotine users, *except at meetings.*" As long as I keep coming to meetings, getting into service, working the steps and keep applying these principles in my life, then I won't fear going back to smoking.

Want to know something? I hope they never find a cure, purely for selfish reasons. If they found a cure, and it would get rid of the physical addition but not the physiological addiction, and I could talk myself into smoking one here and one there, after all, I am not addicted to nicotine anymore. But I put smoke and tar in my lungs, and in time I just might find myself smoking more and more. After all, it still is a mood-altering drug, and we are addicts.

No drug would make my thinking sane. Only God, this Program and the members of NicA does. I like the idea of being addicted, and there is no cure. Why take chances?

GUILT: GOOD TOPIC

False guilt is a wasted emotion. It's a matter of low esteem. My early life was full of false guilt. I was a victim, and naturally, it was always my fault. I did something wrong even if I didn't know what that wrong was. No matter, I fess up I am guilty as charged. LOL.

I would go outside and mediate with a cigarette, and that helped relieve the guilt at least to the point it didn't hurt as much. At least I think it did. I doubt if did, but seemingly it helped.

Real guilt is an honest emotion and a necessary one. "If you feel guilty, then probably you are." Of course, false guilt can come under that saying as well as constructive guilt. Hey, I just made that up. Constructive guilt!

When I feel guilty, that means I did something wrong to somebody, and I need to take action to fix it like an amend. Or maybe it's a feeling that my actions could have been better, and I can take actions not to repeat the same mistakes. If I never felt guilty, then I would never have changed. I thought I didn't need to change anything so that I would go back to my normal life style. Smoke! Ugh!

If I never felt guilty, then I would feel perfect, and I would let you know that too. LOL

As a parent raising four kids, 3 of them were girls; they could be monsters at age 12. But never being a parent before, and not knowing a thing about being a parent, I am going to make mistakes every which way as time goes on. So naturally, I would feel guilty, because I felt I wasn't handling something right. Guilt is what motivates me to do better.

Even false guilt can be a good thing too. Smoking helped me deal with low self esteem. But that false guilt got me to the Program where I could learn what I needed to do. So false guilt can be a motivator too.

If it can make you do better, then bring on the guilt. LOL

HAPPY, JOYOUS & FREE

I never really knew what happy, joyous and free really meant until I quit smoking. Nicotine was the backup drug I used when I didn't want to deal with other issues I hadn't dealt with in AA. It was much easier to smoke the problem away, which BTW really didn't work. I just buried it with all the other things I buried by smoking. I did what I had to do to quit drinking, but I still smoked. I saw others smoking; then, it was the rational thing to do. It was still acceptable in some areas. Even in this day, you can go up to a smoker and bum a smoke. Try and do that going to a bar and asking someone if they will let me sip their beer. You're liable to be thrown out in the street!

Now with that said I had discovered something about my recovery from my drinking and smoking.

I quit smoking before I quit drinking. I have 22 years free of nicotine and 18 years free of alcohol. So how can I say nicotine was my back up drug? I tried quitting alcohol in 1968 and couldn't stay sober until 2003. I was in and out for some time. I did get four years and five years in that time span. And I was smoking like any good smoker would do. I could hide my feelings by smoking and therefore I didn't deal with them, which in its indirect way helped me go out and drink again. I was not dealing with life as I should have. If I couldn't solve my problem through AA, I would use my back up drug, nicotine, and in effect went out drinking again.

Then I quit nicotine and my drinking issues were there, and I had no backup drug. It forced me into sobering up again, and I stayed sober for one day shy of my first year and went back out again. Then I stayed sober for one day beyond my first year and went back out again. And I made another attempt a little more than a year, and in between these bouts of drinking I had to realize if I want to stay nicotine free, I must stop drinking. I began to realize I really wanted some semblance of order in my life. I hit my bottom with alcohol after I hit my bottom with nicotine. I had no backup drugs left to deal with life. Then, I was able to put it all together, and my life changed by really working the 12 Steps in both programs.

In the beginning, I was feeling many bouts of guilt due to the fact I quit smoking before I quit drinking. Just about everyone quit drinking first, then quit smoking. I am doing this recovery wrong. And in time I met several members, not many, but they did the same thing I did. I am a bassackwards guy attempting recovery. LOL

LIVING IN DENIAL?

I did pay attention to the warnings on the pack of cigarettes. I had seen that smoking these cigarettes was unhealthy for me, so I changed to a safer warning. If it said this is bad if you are pregnant or the ones that said smoking causes carbon monoxide, then it was okay to smoke those brands. Was I in denial? Nah. What was wrong with finding a safer cigarette?

I then tried the low tar cigarettes that have holes in the filter. The only problem with them was I couldn't feel like I was smoking with the holy ones. LOL. So after buying a carton of these "holy" cigs, I wrapped the filter with masking tape and then they were okay.

Seeing as that was a lot of work I went back to my old brands even though the warning did suck, but I figured that I had as much chance of dying with the smog in the air as I did smoking—and my family tree all lived smoking and drinking to their mid or late 80's. I had a long way to go. I suppose you could call that denial, but I was looking at it realistically.

You see, I enjoyed my smoking, never mind that I was coughing, different bouts with bronchitis, or walking pneumonia or pleurisy or mild heart problems. I enjoyed feeling that smoke go deep into my lungs, and I could breathe it out into the air making smoke rings and be in heavenly bliss and in that blissful state go into a coughing spasm and coughing up a ton of phlegm and after that take another hit.

Was I living in denial? No, I was smoking the wrong brand. I changed to menthol cigs, and that just made me cough more, so I decided I would change over to pipe smoking. I did that for a while, but when I found out, that can cause throat cancer. I said, "no way Jose, I'm no fool." So I quit the pipe because I didn't want to get throat cancer.

There has to be a way of smoking without getting sick and having everyone on my case. I knew quitting was out of the question. It was too much a part of my life. So I tried rolling my own, but that took too much time. So then I decided to take a hiatus, and I spent my time in the hospital three different times for anywhere from a 5-8 days stretches. On my last trip to the hospital, I was told if I ever come back here and am still smoking that I would be lucky to go home with an oxygen bottle.

Well, it was starting to sink in that I can't do this much longer. So I joined a smoking cessation program and stayed clean for 30 days and told myself I am feeling pretty good so I will have just one and take it from there. Well for the next nine months I was suffering from acute bronchitis 24-7 every day, and how I managed to live, I had no idea. I hurt too bad. I couldn't breathe, and many times I was on my hands and feet coughing and coughing. Each time I coughed, it felt like a knife stabbing me in the chest. I swore I was going to break all my ribs, and finally, I got to the point I didn't care if I lived or died.

This little white piece of paper wrapped around tobacco was causing me all these problems, and I couldn't quit.

I started coming to Nicotine Anonymous, and after going to meetings ten days in a row and on the 11th day, I quit. I wanted to live more than I wanted to die. In fact, I didn't want to die, but I wanted to live. I had no idea what I was going to do, but I quit and haven't found it necessary to pick up another cigarette since then, and that was on 11/21/98, almost 22 and a half years ago. The first year smober was hard, and I call it my "hard walk," but I got through it, and I can say I never want to go through that again. Once is enough for me. When it all comes down to it, I do not have another quit in me. I spent a good 15 years before NicA trying to quit and stay quit, even though I really didn't like the idea of quitting. I still was waiting for a chance to get another hit.

Today I am very grateful I don't smoke and I don't desire one, and it's not part of my life today. Today I am a non-smoker. I don't use the term ex-smoker as it sounds dirty to me.

I have my health back, all things considered. Outside of aging and COPD issues, I am in good health. My heart is in excellent shape for my age, and I enjoy a good night/s sleep almost every night, and that is a bonus. I give all the credit for my smobriety to God and the members of this Program. There is no way I could do this on my own. Heaven only knows I tried many times on my own, only to find myself in another utter failure. Today, I am a clean machine.

Typical Yes Man

I was a typical yes man. I hated disagreement. I went along with anyone because I didn't want to upset the apple cart. I was afraid of being disliked, and I would do anything for approval.

This left me resentful, mad at myself because I didn't have the courage to speak out about what I felt. And to say "NO" was out of the question. I felt like I was useless in the grand scheme of things. So by smoking, I could numb these feelings and get false courage. But that didn't last that long, because it just didn't work anymore. And I sure as hell didn't know how to be honest with myself or others!

It's when I finally gave up smoking for one day at a time, did things start to change. It wasn't easy but do-able, and in working the 12 Steps, it changed my way of doing business with others and myself. When I started to share my feelings in an honest way to the best of my ability for some time, I began to feel good about myself.

I had a long way to go, but it was a start. Every time I got honest, it was one less secret I had to carry. I lived in meetings for a long time, and I truly believed I was a part of the whole. It was a beginning for me to start being of service and I haven't stopped. "The Truth will set you free." Never a truer statement said.

It really feels good these days to say what's on my mind, especially when I know I am going to be in disagreement. I have learned that is the price I have to pay to stand on my convictions. And that feels good, let me tell you.

I am what I am, says Popeye the sailor man. I eat my spinach and speak my mind. I can hold my head up and be proud of it. I do not want that old life back. It got me nowhere but digging the hole I was living in deeper.

I like the idea of "What you see is what you get." I am not perfect, nor do I try to be. I do try to do the best I can. And if I can say that, then everything is okay. I stay in the day and find the day is manageable for me. Asking God for wisdom is a good starter way for solving problems. This program works if you work it, and it won't if you don't. And that is the name of that tune.

HUMOR ME

Humor has to be one of the greatest gifts of life. I have learned that by immersing myself into this program and learning how to deal with life.

I was always an angry, unhappy, and disillusioned guy. I took myself too damn seriously and had nothing to laugh about. Oh, I laughed just to make myself look good to others. I faked funny! I thought I was a victim in the worst way. Now I look back and see I was not unique in this thinking at all.

My first life was birth to entering smobriety. As I enter life my second life, I learn how to deal with life on life's terms, how to solve problems, how to deal with stress, and most importantly, how to laugh at myself. This is a biggie. This shows me that I am not taking myself too seriously. And this keeps me from smoking or even thinking about smoking.

I came home from the store once, and the bag opened up at the bottom, and a dozen eggs hit the floor. I said, "Shoot, well I guess I will clean it up in a bit, and we will have scrambled eggs for dinner. A readymade dinner!" I can always find something humorous about anything, even if it's a sick thought.

I can find something good about anything and something funny about anything. Or I can bitch about what happens and think evil things to do to people who did this to me.

A while back, I turned on the water and nothing, but black water came out. I told my wife, "Hey love, come bring your empty bottles and fill them up and put them in the fridge and we can have cold black water." I have been married for 43 years now, and I can still pull the wool over my wife's eye. She gets mad sometimes, and I laugh my butt off. He-He, I did it again.

This is a crack up: Years ago I went into a pet store to get some pet food for our cats. I picked up a 25 lb. bag of dry food and stood in line. I started a conversation with a fellow behind me, and we were talking about our pets, and I asked him, "Hey have you ever tried eating this pet food? It's dry and tasteful, and it's a good snack." He looked at me and said, "Uh... no." "Well, you should try it. You might like it." And I kept this talk for a few minutes and got some funny looks like I was a nut or something, if they only knew.

I told the cashier maybe they could sell smaller portions for snacks as it is very good. The cashier shook his head. I gave him some money; he gave me my change. I went to my car and sat down laughing my ass off. I never told them I was just joking. I sat in the car and they were shaking their heads. Been back there several times and no one mentions a thing.

Life has its ups and downs. I can learn to accept things, have some fun, and be able to laugh at myself and silly situations.

SPIRITUAL CONNECTION

"Without a connection to my Higher Power, I am the same old person with the same old defects, causing the same old pain in my life and others'."

—A.A. Grapevine

Until I could focus on God and who He is, I would remain who I am. I needed to change. In the beginning, everything I saw, touched, heard, and felt, I needed a cigarette. I couldn't breathe without a thought of a cigarette, and my mind wanted to focus on how a cigarette would make me feel so much better....what a lie that is! And I couldn't even go to the toilet without a smoke. How sick is that?

It was hammered into my head "Do not smoke no matter what even if your ass falls off." If I pick up a smoke, then my head will revert back to where I was before I picked up the cigarette, and then wished that I were back there. Then the trouble begins, because I'm not going to quit, I am going to smoke myself into oblivion. Someday I might try it again. The trap I can fall into with my thinking is very dangerous at times.

It's uncomfortable in the beginning, but I pray to God for the courage to get you through the day and His will. I surrounded myself with NicA members, and at first, lived in meetings night and day. There have been times I almost gave in, but that damn thought of having to start all over again, and giving up my time from being clean kept me going.

At first, I had to learn to accept the cravings as part of my life at the time. They will go away but not overnight. It took me about a year and a half before I could say I lost the obsession to smoke. It just got easier day by day, and the more time I had off cigarettes, the less I wanted to pick one up. I had to keep myself busy, and I would start my day off with prayer, and keep my mind on God and who He is. The more I did that, the more

I learned. Working the Steps made a huge difference in my life. And I said the Serenity prayer many times through the day.

Nothing changes, if nothing changes, and the way is in finding God. I keep this thought in my thinking. That is the true start in getting a spiritual connection.

A difficulty for me was "What am I going to do with my hands?" They were always in the way. I can't sit on them forever. So to relieve that hand to mouth fixation, I drank a lot of water. Every time I had a thought of smoking, I drank water. I kept a bottle of water with me wherever I went. At night, I would place my water on the nightstand, and when I woke up I thought about smoking, I drank water instead. It was a huge help to me.

I cut back on coffee from 3 pots a day to a cup and a half. I needed the caffeine to get me going, but it tasted like crap without a cigarette. Ha-Ha. Then I started to go for a walk in the morning, even before I had my coffee. It was a half mile walk, and I came back. I was energized, and life didn't seem so bad. I kept changing minor routines into other routines, like going to work in different directions for different scenery.

If you're new in your quit, don't give up hope, and keep your eye at the light at the end of the tunnel, and in time you will come out of that tunnel and life will look so much better.

LIFE ON LIFE'S TERMS

Living each day on life's terms was hard in the beginning because I was living life on my terms. When things didn't go my way, which was every day, I had a fit.

It seemed things were always happening to me. Financial crisis, being late for work, customers upset with me, wife mad at me, kids were a pain in the rear, and on and on the list can go. As much as I tried to change these things, it didn't work. Why? Because I put so much self-importance on myself, and it was up to me to fix life. It took a while to realize I am not able to have an answer for everything. God! What a revelation!

I can't fix everything. I realized that smoking wasn't going to fix everything. When I quit, it was like being on the edge of a cliff, and nowhere to go except to keep walking on the edge, or I would fall way down into the rocks below.

So I couldn't smoke, I couldn't deal with life, and I was very unsure what in the hell was going to happen next. The only thing I had going for me was the gentle push God gave me and the program of Nicotine Anonymous.

First, I had to learn how to not smoke for one day, then how to live each day one day at a time. That encompasses dealing with life on life's terms, which is no easy matter in the beginning. Once I had the concept down of living one day at a time, I started to learn to live life on life's terms. Now I see that it is all about acceptance.

I cannot change any circumstance or other people to my point of view, or they should change for my pleasure. When I figured that out, then it became easier. The only thing I can change is myself. Yes, I can change circumstances by making amends. Or I might help with something that is better for all and then leave the rest up to God. I have my opinions and so do others.

I have to realize that my opinion isn't always the best opinion. I must give way to majority rules in any conflict. It sure beats fighting. I fight, I lose—I surrender, I win. I have no control over crises that happen like someone getting sick, someone in the hospital, or an accident or car breakdown, or it rains when I had planned a gathering outside, an appointment gets cancelled, or I lost a job...and the list can go on ad infinitum.

So what can I do in these cases of life on life's terms? I can't change it, I, for the most part, can't fix it, so I have to learn to accept it. Just flow with it, and try to see the other side of the equation. A lot of my "crises" are my own doing. I can prevent these problems by taking care of a potential problem before it happens by being proactive. For example, if I have worn out tires on my car, I replace them before I have a blowout. Or I might save myself a lot of physical problems by keeping appointments and following doctor's suggestions.

Acceptance is the key to all my problems. Acceptance does not mean I have to like what is happening, but to accept it as a fact of life. I pray daily and throughout the day. There is nothing like repeating the Serenity prayer over and over throughout the day to give me a sense of calmness.

"Serenity is not the absence of conflict, but the ability to cope with it." I keep that thought in mind as I go through my day. Don't smoke no matter what and things will change for me. If I smoke, I'm screwed. Blunt and to the point.

It's like cravings. We have to accept those as part of our life at the time we are experiencing them. And as the old saying goes, "This too shall pass." I hated that saying in the beginning. LOL

FIRST 30 DAYS

The first 30 days that I quit was quite boring for me. I sat and watched TV with that thousand yard stare and ate myself into oblivion. I put on 30 lbs. I ran my business okay for the most part, even though it was hard at times. When I got home, I hit the chair and sat there for the rest of the evening staring at the TV and stuffing myself.

By quitting smoking, I found out I had no activities to keep my interest, so I was bored. The only "activity" I had was to light up a cigarette one after another. I could not stay in that dream world. Now I had to find other activities to interest me. Going to meetings every day was quite helpful and kept my eyes on the goal of not smoking. I lived for the meeting every day for 7 days a week. I drove on the average 70 miles round trip to meetings.

Otherwise, I didn't know what to do with myself. The thought of smoking kept coming up, and it seemed like a good idea at times until I thought of about the other side of the coin. I didn't want to return to that hard side of the life of coughing, not breathing, dizzy spells, pain and a general feeling of blah and who gives a damn.

I was and still am a procrastinator. At the beginning of my quit, I found if I made a list of things I needed to do, and did some each day I wasn't as bored. I sensed a feeling of accomplishment. I liked email and writing to others, but sometimes that got too overwhelming. When I let it go and said, "tomorrow," time passes. Finally, I have to grab the bull by the horn and just do it. I find out every time, it wasn't that big of a deal, and I feel so good afterwards. And another day goes by, not smoking.

One of the hardest periods of my quit was when the excitement of not smoking wore off. I was aware the honeymoon was gone, and life of real living hit me. I can't smoke, and I got angry over that. What the hell was I going to do now? I can't smoke, and that pissed me off, and if I smoke, then I will be pissed off. So what the hell was a person going to do? Caught between a hard rock and a hard place. I was told, "This too shall pass," and I wanted to shove that saying up the person's behind who said this. "Yeah, yeah, yeah, this too shall pass and up yours too!

I began to hate this non-smoking crap in a big way because it was not fun. So I began to get into service with little things, but it made me feel important to the group and helped me not think of smoking for a bit. I became a treasurer for two groups, and as time went on I became a secretary of another group. This helped me to be happy about being a non-smoker. I never say ex-smoker as that is a dirty word to me. I am a non-smoker. Those first few months were hell on wheels, and as I look back on hindsight, I am glad it was hard because I do not want to ever go back and have to do this same crap all over again. I earned my time free of nicotine, and it is precious to me.

I was told the day would come when you realize you really haven't thought about smoking. And I said bull crap! That will never happen. And it did! About four months or so after I quit, I was closing my business the thought came to me that I didn't think about smoking. I mean like Wow! This was a big thing for me.

And my journey of recovery began like wildfire. And over the years, it has paid off a lot of dividends. I am alive and well and love living life on life's terms. I am in better health than I ever was. I have a lot of freedom to do or not do whatever I want — my choice. I don't have to make excuses any more. I learn to accept things I do as my responsibility, good or bad.

And so as another day passes, I feel pretty good. And now I will take it easy.

FAITH AND TRUST

The trouble with us addicts, speaking for myself, is the realization I can't see what is going to happen tomorrow, or even for that matter the next second. I don't have a clue. But I'm supposed to at least get "along" with other people, work, spend money, pay bills, go places, learn a trade, etc.

Because of my smoking and drinking issues, I was a mess, and it didn't matter what I did, it turned out crappy to my way of thinking.

Throughout my growing up years, I was taught the God of the Bible (which I believe BTW), but my senses weren't relaying that info to me. I couldn't see God, I couldn't hear God, I couldn't feel God, so how am I going to believe in God? This ghostly apparition is among us, and if He is, how can He talk and guide all 7.5 billion people in the world? That was just too much to believe in.

I kept that thought with me for some time while still smoking. I knew God existed, but what kind of God is He? I smoked myself into a shriveled old nutcase, while I was digging my grave and putting the shovel down and ready to jump in the grave I dug for myself. This was very "rational thinking" indeed. Ha!

But this is an illusion! I can see God by what He has created. I have a common sense that tells me this whole world didn't just happen, and all things didn't just all of a sudden appear, and out of nowhere, start this life process without something or someone creating it.

All of a sudden, at this moment, I wanted to live, not die. It was a strong feeling. When I quit, I literally had to adapt to a new lifestyle that was foreign to me, but I also knew whatever I did or thought was a bunch of BS and nothing else worked.

Enter Nicotine Anonymous and their premise to believe in a Higher Power in order to change into a non-smoker who is happy not to smoke. This is a spiritual program, and I don't take it lightly.

There are seven Steps that refer to God. Steps 2, 3 5 6, 7, 11, and 12.

Take those Steps away, and I am left with Steps 1, 4, 8, 9, and 10. Can you imagine admitting I am an addict, and I must write an inventory and make a list of who I hurt and make amends to them and then take a daily inventory and be ready to admit when I'm wrong? There is no damn way I would even think about doing those things.

There is no answer or relief for me in a 5 step program. So I would leave and continue on my "merry" way. How many times have you heard someone say to leave the spiritual part out of this Program and just teach me how not to smoke? "I don't need God, because I can do things by myself, I am self-sufficient you see." If that is the case, why am I so screwed up? Pride goes before a fall. And my pride was up there on the top of it all.

I came to Nicotine Anonymous and went to a meeting every night for 90 days. Those first ten days, I argued the merits of the program and everything else. However, I couldn't get away from what I have seen: many members with multiple years still coming to meetings. They were very happy and they all talked about God. Hmmmmm.

At this point in my life I believed in the God of the Bible, but I felt He had failed me and wasn't all cracked up to be what was said about God. I had the faith but not the trust. For some time before I came to NicA, I prayed to God to take the desire to smoke away from me, and then I will quit smoking. That never happened! This was even too big for God to do. So I dumped Him. Not realizing I am praying a foxhole or conditional type of prayer.

Then I had a moment of enlightenment. I was at a meeting, and the discussion was on the Third Step. I made my stupid comments, and after the meeting, someone told me, "Gary, why don't you just give up?" That made more sense to me at that moment than anything else. I was a fighter and was always losing. So why fight then? Give up and win.

And then on the 11th day of coming to NicA, I quit smoking on November 21, 1998. Praise God I haven't thought of smoking for so many years now! And it feels good not to be enslaved by that stupid piece of crap I put in my mouth and inhaled, and that smoke that burned my insides up. I lived the lie that smoking helped me cope with life. If that was true, why would I want to fall over a 2nd story business complex and end it all? And meanwhile, wanting a cigarette at the same time. insanity!

I had to re-energize my faith and trust in a power whom I call God. Faith is one thing, but trust is another thing all by its self. There is a story of a man who walked across the canyon from one side to the other on a rope while he was pushing a wheelbarrow. He did this every day for sport. After a while, one person there asked another person, "Do you think he can do it again?" The other person said yes, "I have the faith he can." That is faith, but trust is getting into the wheelbarrow — a whole new concept.

Sometimes when I have to trust God, it's unsettling, but I go forward, and God does come through. It's over many times of God coming through that my trust is built up again and again. By working these 12 Steps of trusting, it gets easier to trust God, myself and others as time goes on. The saying that "You don't need the ticket until the train gets here," is nerve wracking. "Hey God, can you give me a little leeway here?" LOL

Faith and trust are like a light bulb. Let's say I've never seen a light switch and someone says if I flip that light switch the light will come on.

And I say, "Sure it will." And it does, and after many times seeing this I have the faith it will come on if I flip the light switch.

Trust is believing in the unknown. We place ourselves in a trustful mode when it comes to things we like and need. For example: computers, TV, microwaves and lighting.. All this has happened because of the theory of electricity. It wasn't possible until the theory was put into practice.

So it is with God. I could say it is a theory of His being here, but I have to step out in faith to see that it works and after I get the faith, I had to step out on trust in a very uncomfortable situation in my life. And God came through.

Do you know something? If I turn my life over to God and learn to pray, then I find I have a lot more time to do things I have worries about a whole lot of nothing. It's God's problem. At least this works for me. Today I have faith and trust that God does exist and cares for me and my family. End of story!

OBSESSION WITH SMOKE

When I came to NicA, I had no idea of what to expect. All I knew for sure was I had to quit smoking, or I will die right in front of you. The idea of quitting smoking scared the crap out of me. I knew that it was impossible to keep a quit, but the idea of not ever having another cigarette was something that I couldn't conceive of either. I wanted to smoke, and I wanted not to smoke, and neither option sounded good to me. I was stuck between a hard rock and a hard place.

Yes, it was hard, and that's an understatement! But it did get better as long as I didn't pick up. The cravings or mental obsession did not go away for some time. It was a year and a half before I could say the obsession to smoke left me. I found new things to do that made me enjoy my new life without my old "friend."

Until I quit, I either never knew or had forgotten the joys of breathing—not coughing, not being woozy. I could eat better, I didn't stink, and people didn't give me a dirty look. Nobody preached to me.. Finally, after many, many years, I found my new home, a place I had been searching for a long time. Nicotine Anonymous was my new home.

I have been in NicA for over 22 years, and you're not going to get rid of me. So there!! I never want to have to quit again. I'm glad it was hard because it stays with me. I worked harder to stay clean and fought to quit listening to my head spouting off how hard it is not to smoke, "Light one sucker, and you will feel better. Nobody really appreciates the hell you're going through, so screw everyone, smoke baby, smoke. You haven't had a cigarette for a week now, so give yourself a break. Reward yourself. This quitting stuff is too hard and too boring. I need that relaxation a good smoke gives me." And on and on, my head went.

"Hey Gary, light up, and you will feel better."

"Oh yeah, how many years ago was that?"

"Go ahead and have one."

"Not today, sucker. Maybe tomorrow"

"Hey, you can't function without a cigarette."

"I don't know about that, but I do know I will die if I smoke."

This voice that was in my head way a strong feeling established over 49 years of smoking.

I had to learn not to listen to my head and counter attack it with positive statements.

So I quit and I expected that the voice should go away in a few days. That was a lie. As long as it resided in my head while smoking, you best believe the voice would reside in my head for a long time. That's the nature of the beast. I had to accept that as a fact and move on from there.

I had to stay connected, go to meetings, not give up the idea of quitting, and pray to the God of my understanding for help not to smoke. Just for today only--the hell with tomorrow.

This program works if you work it—but it won't if you don't.

A HARD NUT TO CRACK

The creation of a thousand forests is in one acorn.

—Ralph Waldo Emerson

Before the forests can grow, the acorn has to be planted, watered and cared for a long time, one day at a time. So it is with recovery. Even with all this time in recovery, I didn't get free overnight.

How did that work? It took a lot of action to get from a scared, angry, lonely, person dying from smoking. I was shy and inhibited, and I lived different personas to fit the occasions in my life.

I am a more authentic person these days. Yes sometimes I fear, and that is normal, but I move forward in spite of my fear. Today, I am not afraid of being who I am. I like myself very much and that is a huge biggie for me. I can speak my opinions even if everyone disagrees with me, that's okay too. I am always available to learn something new.

When I was quitting, the first thing I had to do was admit I was powerless over nicotine. It controlled my life. When the addiction spoke, I smoked. I had no say so in the matter. Until I admitted I am utterly powerless over this drug and under no circumstances can I smoke, then and then only I felt I had a chance.

I went to meetings and heard others. In time I began to listen to suggestion and took them, applied them to my life. This went on day by day, week by week, month by month. I learned a little about myself and what to do each day. I slowly, but surely got myself immersed in the Program, and then into service, so I could give it away, and forget about myself. That was a good feeling. I had a lot of changing to do each and every day. A little here and a little there added up as time went on. I applied these 12 Steps in my life, and it has been a miraculous recovery for me.

My first year off nicotine I call my "hard walk," but I was so determined not to pick up, that it reaped rewards for me health-wise, as well as emotionally and spiritually. The one thing I kept in my head is "Do not smoke no matter what, even if my ass falls off." There was no reason for me to smoke. The reasons to smoke were all excuses, and there were many of them. If I could find a justifiable reason to smoke, I might have picked up. The only reason I could find to smoke was the fact I smoked because I am addicted to nicotine.

So if I realize I can't smoke, then that reason was good enough. It was a good reason not to smoke. After almost 22 years free of nicotine, I have not found a reason to smoke. So it's reasonable to say I won't have a problem today with regard to smoking. I have had to work hard at it, and that was good for me. I learned to trust God, did my inventory, made amends, have been of service to help others.

It was a battle I fought, and a battle I wanted to win. The fruits are that I did win the battle on a day-by-day basis. I am not saying I won't ever have a problem dealing with wanting a cigarette, but I doubt it very much. It's been years since I have wanted one. I have lost my obsession and desire to smoke. That is a biggie. A gift from God

And now I practice these principles I have learned in all my affairs. That is a mandatory thing for me to do. That's the 12th Step in action. If I do not work the 12th Step, and I worked the other 11 Steps, then it's all for naught. *I cannot keep it if I do not give it away!*

By giving it away, I can truthfully say I have no fear of smoking for today! And that's all that counts. I planted the acorn, I watered it, I pruned it and took good care of it, and I grew from it into what I am today.

AVERTING GREATER PAIN

I know for me when I was smoking, I just let things go as it was too painful to do them. So I did what I thought was enjoyable...Smoke. And when I did do something, I would feel good about it and do some more and would get tired. Enough is enough today. "I need to relax and have a smoke."

And would sit on my butt and let things go and was once again back where I started. It always finished with a smoke. What a rat race. It made me feel useless, and I had to have a smoke over that.

For me, I got sick and tired of being sick and tired and was reaching the point I had to quit smoking. Can't say I like the idea of not smoking, but I had to or die. God took me out of where I was and put where I am today. It wasn't an easy transition, yet it's been a worthwhile change in life. Wherever there is change, there is pain.

The pain of doing something now to avert a greater pain—of smoking myself to death—is a much better strategy. But for this to happen, I had to reach the bottom where I was willing to do anything I had to do to not smoke. And I am glad I did! I learn from my experiences not by osmosis. I have to take action.

DEEP BREATHING

Taking that deep breath really helps me slow down and realize what I'm doing. It's a normal kind of action I take on a daily basis. Deep breathing helps me to think better and not run on my emotions. It slows me down from walking 10 miles an hour to two miles an hour.

This happened to me many years ago, but it stayed with me till now:

I was in my computer room (and that was when I had one--lol), and my truck was parked up the hill a ways. Suddenly, I desperately needed something out of the truck. I ran out of the house to go get it as it was *soooooooo* important that I have it *noooooooow!* I got to the edge of my garage, stopped, and grabbed the corner of the building and said, "What in the hell am I doing?"

I slowly counted to ten and then did some deep breathing exercises. I walked very slowly to my truck, got what I wanted, and slowly walked back to the house at a snail's pace, and did what I had to do whatever it was. Whatever it was, it got done within 15 minutes or so. Nothing like being on a roller coaster going nowhere fast!

I have to catch myself and tell myself to slow down because the world isn't coming to an end.

SMOKING DREAMS

I remember one smoking dream that scared the living crap out of me. I woke up realizing I had gone back to smoking, and everyone in my family knew I was smoking again. They were royally upset with me for the umpteenth time. I had been going to NicA meetings regularly for a few weeks, and I didn't know what I should do. Do I cop out about smoking or lie about it? I knew I was "letting everyone down," and I didn't know what to do. I was the biggest loser in town.

I laid in bed for a couple of minutes kicking myself in the behind, and got up and went to the bathroom and then brushed my teeth and I was looking in the mirror, and the thought came to my mind. IT WAS ONLY A DREAM! A good 3-4 minutes went by before I realized it was only a dream…OMG! And then I became very grateful that I wasn't smoking. I didn't know what grateful was until I had that dream. I was in such an emotional turmoil over that dream. It was so real and vivid.

And then I had a funny smoking dream later on. I was dreaming I was at a NicA meeting and after the meeting, I wanted everyone to come outside to my car, because I had a gift for everyone that was at the meeting. So they all came outside and got behind me, and I opened the trunk of my car, and it was loaded with cartons of Marlboro cigarettes. I started to hand out cartons to everyone. I heard this one voice who was very instrumental in keeping me smober, and she said, "Garrrrrrrrrrreeeee! What the hell are you doing?" And I woke up. I shook my head, and thought, "My God, how stupid these dreams can be!"

One dream several years ago really got to me. I had a smoking dream, and I woke up and went back to sleep. Damn if I didn't have a drinking dream! What the hell is this about? So I managed to go back to sleep, and I woke up again with a smoking dream. Now I have to tell you that really bothered me. I got up and stayed up as I was afraid to go back to sleep. That feeling stayed with me for a couple of days. All I remember is I had something heavy on my mind when I went to bed. I don't remember now what it was, nor if it was important.

I still have smoking dreams about once a year. I call them my annual dreams. It doesn't bother me in the least. I wake up and tell myself; it's just another dream. I go back to sleep and forget all about for a couple of days. Then, when it comes back to me, I remember. To analyze these dreams is a waste of time to me. I have no control over what my sub-conscience says to while I am asleep. If nothing else it's probably the mood I went to bed with. Since I have 49 years of smoking thoughts in my head, sometime it is bound to come out in a dream!

LIES OF INSANE THINKING

After I was about nine months clean from nicotine, I was in Colorado to be with my wife and their family reunion. The elevation was over 8500 feet, and that is definitely not good for my COPD, but I figured, I can tough it out since I quit smoking. I would just take it easy.

We were in a park having a BBQ, and I was walking to the restroom. I just simply fell down flat on my face. I could not breathe. The very first thought that came to mind was that I needed a cigarette to help me breathe.

That is truly insane thinking. I also believed that smoking relieved my stress.

Well, that's a lie too. In a sense, it did make me feel more relaxed, but really all it did was relieve the craving for another hit. So I guess I could say it did relieve the anxiety. I believed it made me think better, but that too was a lie. Smoking just gave me more time to be with my friend, "niccababy." I could fantasize all kinds of over the top ideas that never came to fruition. I could think how good the cigarette was to me and how good it tasted—I was living a lie.

It tasted like s#*t, so who was I kidding? It must have been that fat elephant in the living room that was telling me that.

I began to think about how bad the tar and other stuff that I was putting into my body, and what it was doing to me. So instead of quitting smoking, I bought a carton of Nows. Those were the low tar cigarettes that had holes all around the filter. That was like sucking in air. So as not to let these cigarettes go to waste, I spent a lot of time wrapping scotch tape around the filter so I could get a "normal" hit. Insanity. What I wouldn't do to protect my "friend" and all the work I put behind the act of smoking. The sneaking out, the lies, the money spent, the medical bills in hospitals and doctor offices, not to mention all the cough syrup that I bought.

I spent a lot of money on cigarettes over the years I smoked, but I really believe I spent more money on medical costs, burnt car seats, burnt furniture, burnt clothing not to mention how many days I have taken off work for one reason or another — plagued with bronchitis, walking pneumonia and just a general feel of the f-its. Add it all up, and it's worse than the national debt. Well, maybe not quite but you get the picture.

STEP TWELVE

> Step Twelve: Having had a spiritual awakening as the result
> of these steps, we tried to carry this message to nicotine
> users and to practice these principles in all our affairs.

Quick doesn't stick. This is a lifelong way of life we practice the rest of our lives one day at a time.

I used nicotine for 49 years, and I used to think because I quit for a short time like a month all things would be hunky dory. This new life in recovery from nicotine addiction is a new norm. It takes some time to get used to. I lied and cheated all my life—do you think I am going to have this overnight success of a personality change and everyone will notice how good I am these days? Ha! I had to learn to do the next right thing for a long, long time before it became comfortable for me. Then others noticed too. The key word for me is practice. Strive for perfection, and that comes with practice. That is the striving thing, not perfection.

This is where the Twelve Steps come into play. They're meant to show me the error of my ways and how to change it. And then I go out in the world and practice what I have learned. I cannot be one way here online or at a meeting and be somebody else outside these perimeters of safety. I have to try to be the same way at work, play and at home at all times. Or it means nothing.

I go to meetings, I am in service, I sponsor off and on, I try to do the next right thing. When I don't, I usually recognize it at the time, and I make the necessary amends. That is the Tenth Step in action. Do I just work these steps one time only? Heaven forbid no! The principles of the Program are intertwined in my life, woven throughout my life. When something isn't right, I have an intuitive thought about what to do to correct it.

So do I screw up? All the time. Day by day, I learn how to live each day to the best of my ability. For me, what works best for me is to be in service wherever I can. Yes, at times it gets tiresome, but I benefit from it. My problems become petty when I am helping someone else. I don't become a victim. Trust me, I know all about being a victim. Staying involved helps me not to regret the past, not to forget it, but not regret it. After all, it is part of my life. If I had no past, then who would I be? I might as well be in a coma.

As long as I try and do the next right thing each day or each moment, then I have to figure God has control over my being, or I wouldn't be doing the next right thing. My previous behavior would be to see how I can hurt you or cheat you.

Today, I get into tempting situations, and I have to ask myself, "What would God do in this case?" The answer comes quickly. Sometimes it's the hard thing to do, but it's the easiest way once it's done. And I feel good about my decision. Things work out for the good for the most part. Yes, life sucks at times, and that's where acceptance comes into play. I can't change people, places or things. No matter how hard I try, it ends up in a dismal failure.,

I can change only myself, and that's all I have to do. An amazing thing happens when I only clean up my side of the street. The other side comes around to my way of thinking, and we all get along with each other.

WHAT HAVE I MISSED SINCE I QUIT?

What have I missed since I quit? I am not coughing; I am not wheezing, I don't have yellow fingers, I don't have many back pains, I don't have any headaches, I am keeping my blood where it belongs instead of coughing it up. I smell better; people like to be around me,

I am not so nervous, I am not full of anxiety, not worrying about a lot of things. I sleep like an angel however an angel sleeps...ha-ha. I eat well—all the junk food I can find—as well as decent meals. I haven't lost any weight or gained any over the years. I enjoy living. I enjoy each day as it comes. I don't have any desire to pick up and haven't for many, many years.

I deal with life on life's terms by acceptance or change which every works best. I don't really get angry anymore like I used to. I was a raging lunatic, and thank God cigarettes helped deal with my anger and life—is that denial? I try not to live in denial, I look for real solutions now, and that works great. Since I quit, life is good for this ole" pea picker.